Techniques in VALVULAR HEART SURGERY

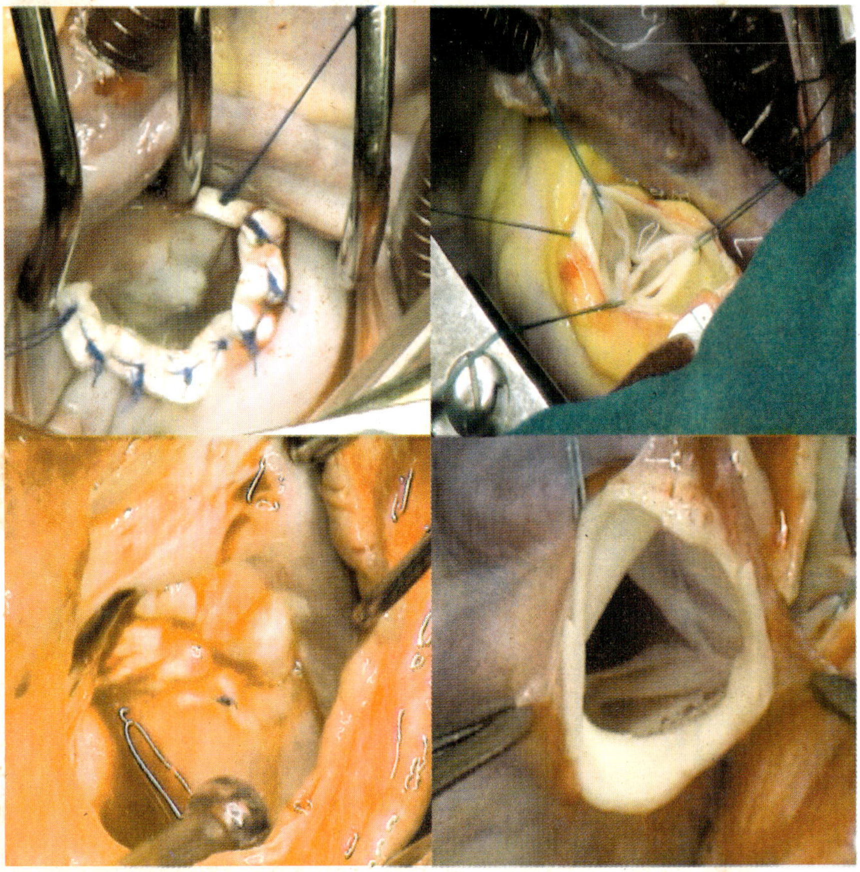

Techniques in VALVULAR HEART SURGERY

A. SAMPATH KUMAR
Professor
Department of Cardiothoracic and Vascular Surgery
All India Institute of Medical Sciences, New Delhi

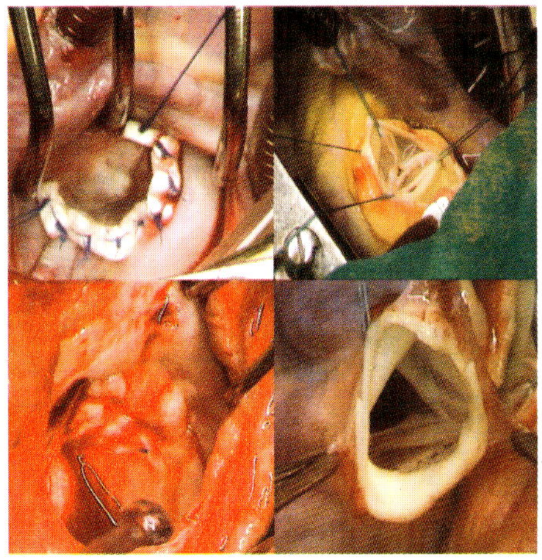

CBS
CBS PUBLISHERS & DISTRIBUTORS
NEW DELHI • BANGALORE

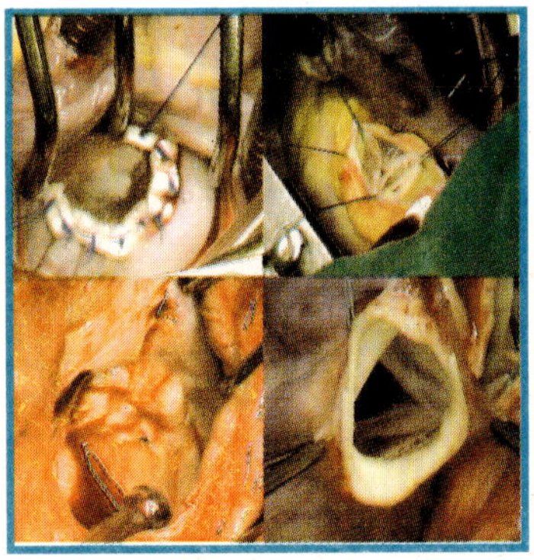

Techniques in
VALVULAR
HEART SURGERY

ISBN: 81-239-1486-5

First Edition: 2007

Published by :
Satish Kumar Jain for CBS Publishers & Distributors,
4596/1-A, 11 Darya Ganj, New Delhi - 110 002 (India)
E-mail : cbspubs@vsnl.com
Website : www.cbspd.com

Production Director : Vinod K Jain

Branch Office :
Seema House, 2975, 17th Cross, K.R. Road,
Bansankari 2nd Stage, Bangalore - 560070
Fax : 080-26771680 • E-mail : cbsbng@vsnl.net

Typeset at :
CBS P&D Typesetting Unit

Printed at :
Swastik Packagings, Delhi-110 092

*to
my
parents,
teachers,
students
and
patients*

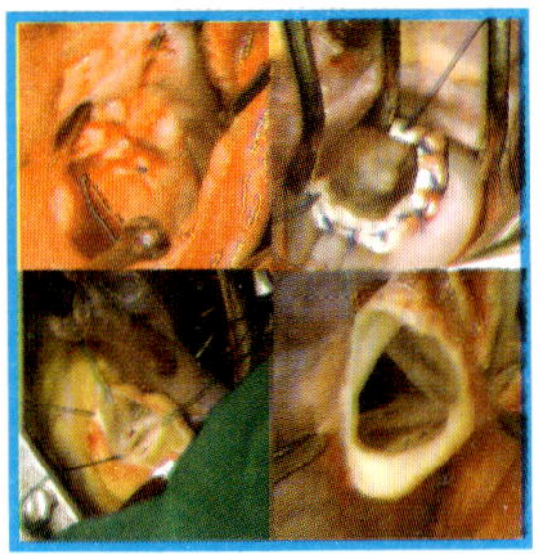

Preface

I considered writing this book when I observed that my students and colleagues were having considerable difficulty in performing these operations. A cardiac surgeon's training begins with valvular heart surgery, almost everywhere. I have taught many surgeons. Almost all of them had the basic skills which they were unable to harness for this purpose. I learnt surgery the hard way, as my teacher put it. He said he could hold my hand and teach me or throw me in the jungle and watch me survive. I survived. I find myself using both techniques with my own students. For some who are shy and fear the consequences I will hold their hand and guide them through every step. For some others there is need only to supervise. Tell them where they are likely to falter in their steps. In any case three decades of exclusive cardiac surgical experience has taught me that the basic or fundamental characteristics of a surgeon are the essential ingredients for success. These are:

(a) **Eye of an eagle** — where visual perception absorbs most of the technical aspects of surgery,

(b) **Hands of woman** — nimble fingers that become dextrous enough to make surgery look simple and easy to perform, and

(c) **Heart of a lion** — courage and fortitude to accomplish a goal that you have thought of.

Without these simple and yet very vital attributes surgeons become mere technicians. These attributes separate the craftsman from the technician. I learnt the "art of surgery" from someone who created new coronary arteries. He did not do just bypasses like others. It is these attributes I intend to teach through the text and illustrations in this monograph.

A comprehensive text that illustrates clearly all the currently available techniques in valvular heart surgery seems to be a need of the hour. One may find each of these techniques familiar from journal articles already published. However, this provides a ready reference with illustrations on the steps of an operation that can be glanced at, just before performing one. It will also help the novice (the rookies) in cardiac surgery to hone their skills and acquire the speed and efficiency that is so vital for a successful outcome. I sincerely hope that by sharing my personal experience, I would help many surgeons in performing these operations and their patients in enjoying quality service.

There are, of course, limitations that are inherent in any technical manual. Some of the complicated procedures in valvular surgery are omitted either because they are now relegated to history or new and better techniques are currently in use. I welcome your suggestions for improvements in the text, illustrations and any other lacunae you may find. I will endeavour to fulfill these in the subsequent revisions of this book.

I have dealt with each valve separately. This is done for convenience both for the reader and the writer. There is no doubt in my mind that in cardiac surgery one cannot ignore the interrelationships of the various valves. For example, severe aortic regurgitation can produce pathological abnormalities of a normally functioning mitral valve. The surgeon, however, cannot afford to ignore these or residual lesions that are sometimes as fatal as the original disease.

I sincerely hope the readers will find this book readable, understandable and applicable in their practice.

A. Sampath Kumar
Professor
Department of Cardiothoracic and Vascular Surgery
All India Institute of Medical Sciences
New Delhi

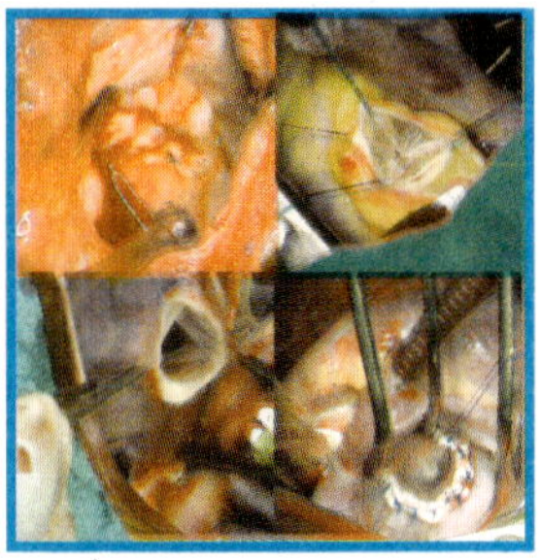

Techniques in Valvular Heart Surgery

This is a textbook in the area of heart surgery, a superspecialty subject. The book clearly describes the special technical steps of operation for heart valve surgery. A book of this nature which concentrates only on one aspect of heart surgery is not available. Books on heart surgery techniques describe only a few of the procedures stepwise. However, this particular book describes all surgical procedures for all human heart valve diseases. Some of these techniques have not been described in any textbook so far. These special techniques have evolved only at the All India Institute of Medical Sciences and in the author's experience.

The book has a descriptive text interspersed with colour photographs and line drawings illustrating the photographs. The text has been well supplemend by a DVD Rom containing video clips of the selected surgical procedures.

The book is useful for students of cardiovascular surgery, cardiothoracic surgeons, medical college libraries, and industries which produce products for these operations.

Dr. A. Sampath Kumar

is a Professor at the Department of Cardiothoracic and Vascular Surgery, All India Institute of Medical Sciences, New Delhi, India, since 1992. He has 35 years of experience and has performed 10,000 heart surgeries for valvular problems so far. This textbook primarily describes the techniques used by him in these operations.

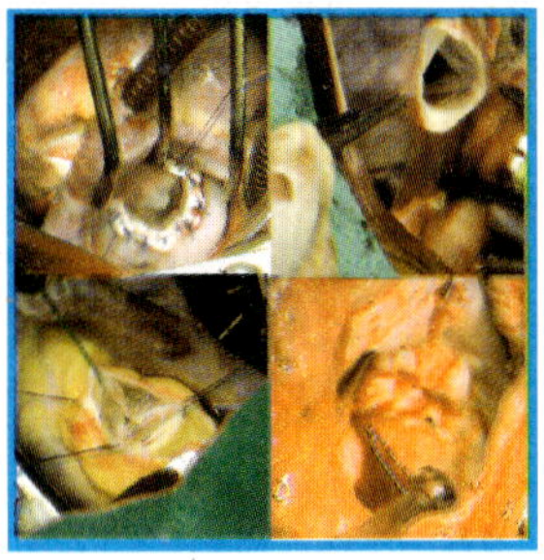

Acknowledgements

Techniques in cardic valve surgery described in this textbook were mastered over three decades and in thousands of patients. This is a tribute to all those patients who reposed their trust in my skills and permitted me to enter and learn from their hearts.

I could not have reached here without the blessings, encouragement and training I have received from a large number of teachers in India and abroad at the undergraduate, postgraduate and at the superspecialty levels. I shall ever remain grateful to all of them.

Behind the success of this monograph is a constant encouragement and support from my family. My wife Pamela, daughter Ratna and son Ananth deserve my sincere gratitude.

Teaching has always been a very satisfying function. It is successful only when there is someone who wishes to learn. I am indebted to my colleagues, students, nurses, operation theatre staff, perfusionists and physiotherapists.

Cardiac surgery is a team effort and here my tributes go out to my colleagues from cardiology, cardiac radiology, cardiac pathology and cardiac anesthesiology.

I must thank my staff, particularly Ms Mini Varghese and Ms Sanju Guleria, for their sincere efforts to transform my manuscript into a readable form. I am grateful to Mr Stephen Marazzi for the superb line drawings. I must thank the editors of *Texas Heart Institute Journal* and the *Indian Journal of Thoracic and Cardiovascular Surgery* for permission to reproduce some illustrations, which have been duly acknowledged in the text.

Finally, I am thankful to Mr YN Arjuna, Publishing Director, CBS Publishers & Distributors, who took up this project with all sincerity and enthusiasm.

A. Sampath Kumar

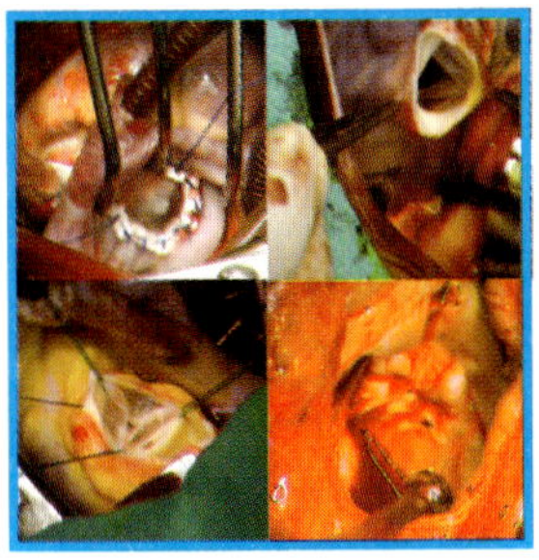

Contents

Techniques in VALVULAR HEART SURGERY

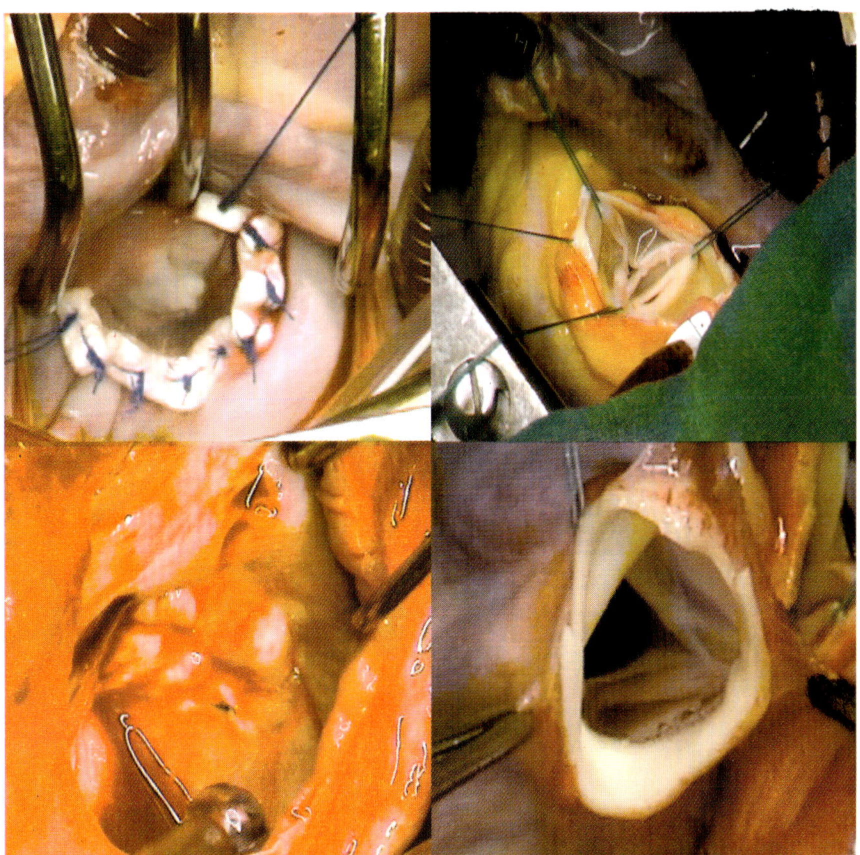

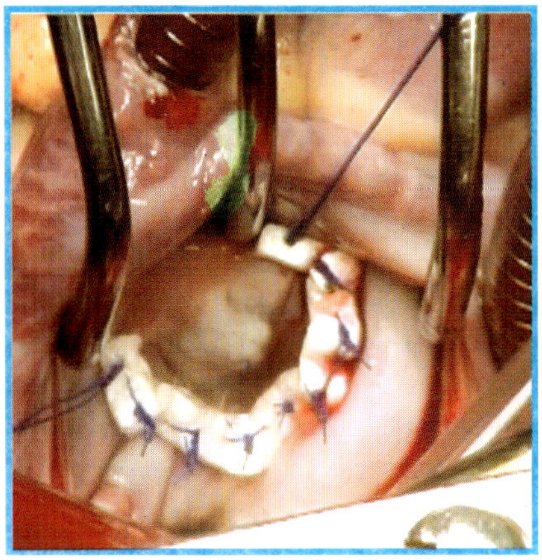

1

The Mitral Valve

ANATOMY

So named because of its resemblance to a Bishop's *mitre*, this complex structure continues to elude the scientists and surgeons in finding a suitable substitute. It is the most commonly affected valve in the human heart. Although it is not certain why, it is believed that the mitral valve is affected more often because it closes against the highest pressure (the left ventricular systolic pressure) in the human heart.

The mitral apparatus comprises the annulus, cusps, chordae and papillary muscles. The left atrium and left ventricle complete the other functional elements. The anterior leaflet has blood flowing on both sides; from the left atrium on its inlet side and from left ventricle to aorta on its outlet side. When seen in a closed position, the commissural closure line resembles a 'smile'.

This design has remained virtually unchanged for over four million years. However, each mitral valve is as individual in appearance as the face of the person who owns it. Many have described this valve as having three to seven cusps, commissures, etc. For surgical purposes this valve has two well recognised and identifiable cusps. A complete anatomical description of the mitral valve can be found in the publications referred to at the end of this chapter.

PHYSIOLOGY

In the living, the mitral valve is dynamic. It changes its shape, size and appearance during the cardiac cycle to allow free and unobstructed flow from the left atrium in diastole; and support for the ventricular systole and opening up of the left ventricular outflow tract in the ejection period of left ventricular systole. It can increase its effective orifice area from 2.5 cm^2 at rest to 5.5 cm^2 at peak exercise. The subvalvular apparatus with continuity from annulus to papillary muscle and ventricular wall provides the scaffold for normal ventricular function and prevents undue dilatation of the left ventricle. The anterior flexion of the annulus provides easy coaptation and expansion of the left ventricular outflow diameter in left ventricular systole. Even at peak exercise gradients of no more than 2–3 mm Hg can be measured in the normal human mitral valve.

METHODS OF STUDY

Currently echocardiography (M mode, two-dimensional, Doppler, colour flow) provides the most comprehensive, visual and dynamic assessment of the mitral valve function. It is noninvasive, reliable and repeatable. Valve area, gradients and quantification of regurgitant flows can all be measured noninvasively. In addition, assessment of valve morphology, reparability and surgical outcome on the table can be performed by transoesophageal echocardiography. This is easy to learn and use, and extends the surgeon's perception of the valve in its dynamic state. There are few indications, if any, for catheterization and angiocardiography is required mostly for elderly patients suspected to have coronary artery lesions as well.

MITRAL STENOSIS

Mitral stenosis is nearly always caused by rheumatic heart disease. A rare congenital deformity causes mitral stenosis and is known as parachute mitral valve. In rheumatic heart disease (chronic) the valve cusps become thickened, rolled up and contracted. The chordae are thick and fused. Contraction of the chordae pulls up the papillary muscles up to the cusps. The commissures begin to fuse at the annulus and extend towards the centre ultimately causing severe narrowing of the valve orifice. From 3.5 cm^2 it may reduce to 0.5 cm^2 (critical mitral stenosis). Atrial fibrillation may develop due to elevated left atrial pressure and in such patients a thrombus may form in the atrial appendage or the atrial cavity. In long standing mitral stenosis the valve cusps/chordae may calcify. Extensive calcification can extend to the annulus or the ventricular muscle.

SURGICAL TREATMENT

Indications

Symptomatic patients with mitral stenosis will need mitral valvotomy. This operation was first performed by Bailey and Harken in 1948. Closed mitral valvotomy is indicated in patients with symptomatic, isolated, noncalcific mitral stenosis, and in normal sinus rhythm.

In patients with atrial fibrillation, preoperative assessment should be done by transesophageal echocardiography. If a thrombus is absent, they may undergo a closed mitral valvotomy after 6 weeks of oral anticoagulation. If a thrombus is seen, an open mitral commissurotomy is the best option.

Closed Mitral Valvotomy

Anticoagulants are discontinued 48 hr before surgery. General endotracheal anaesthesia with ECG and noninvasive blood pressure monitoring are sufficient. The patient is placed in right semilateral position with a sandbag under the left scapula and one under the buttocks. The left hand is placed over the patient's head. Skin presentation is form right midclavicular line to the spine posteriorly, from the axilla to the umbilicus below.

A curvilinear incision is made over the fifth left intercostal space. In women the incision is made 1 cm below and parallel to the breast-fold. The incision is deepened and the pleural space entered through the fifth intercostal space. The pleural incision is extended anteriorly and posteriorly avoiding the internal mammary artery. A rib spreader or retractor is placed in the intercostal space and opened to provide adequate exposure.

A large sponge is placed between the pericardium and the left lung and the lung is retracted with a malleable retractor.

The left phrenic nerve over the pericardium is identified. The pericardium is held with artery forceps 1 cm anterior to the left phrenic nerve and opened. This incision is extended down to the level of the diaphragm and upwards over the main pulmonary artery. Here the thymus requires to be freed in young patients. The free edge of the pericardium is pulled up to the drape with 4–6 stay sutures (Figs 1.1, 1.2). A diastolic thrill is palpable over the left ventricle and the left atrial appendage is usually enlarged. In patients with atrial fibrillation the left atrial appendage may be shrunken.

The left atrial appendage is gently palpated for a thrombus. It is then held with the forceps and a clamp is placed just above the junction with the left atrium. An incision is made in the left atrial appendage. The incision is extended to about 2 cm in length with the Pott's scissors freeing all musculae pectinati. The 4-0 silk (or braided) sutures are used for stay sutures, three on each side and held on haemostats (Figs 1.3, 1.4).

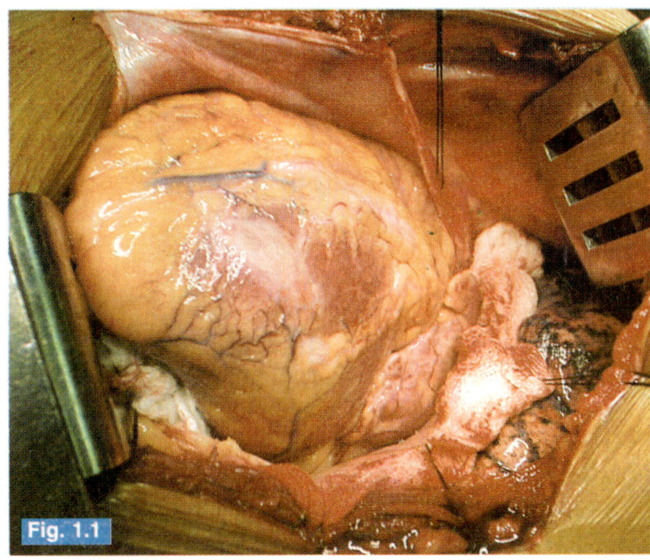

Fig. 1.1

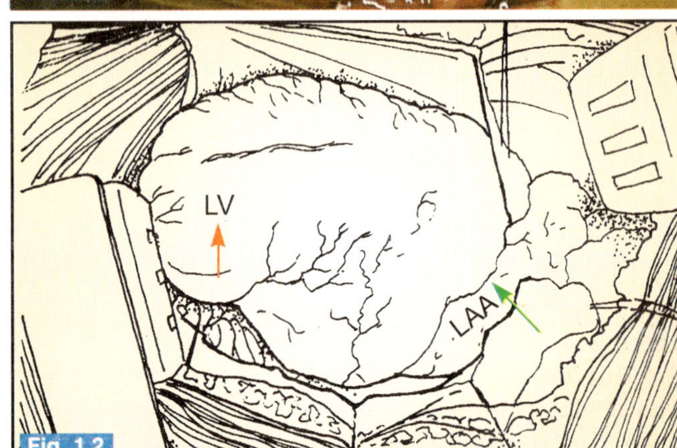

Fig. 1.2

Figs 1.1, 1.2: Exposure of the heart through a left anterior thoracotomy. The pericardium is opened. LAA left atrial appendage, LV left ventricle.

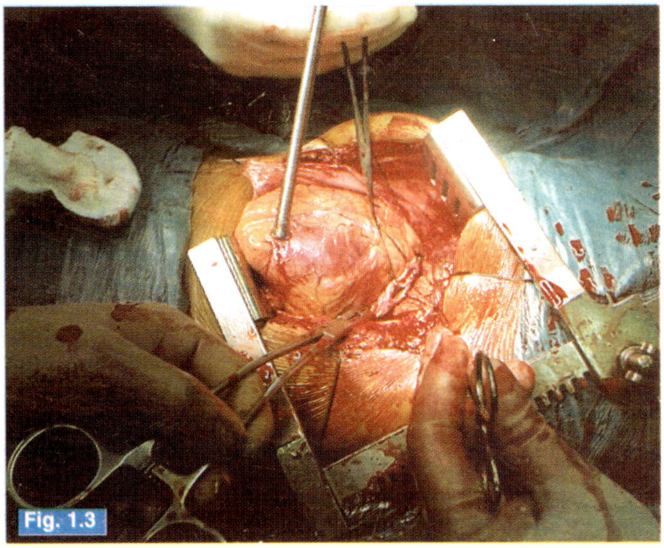

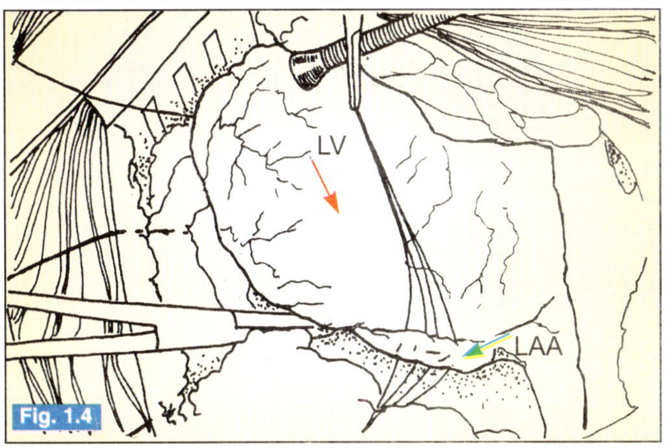

Figs 1.3, 1.4: Closed mitral valvotomy. The left atrial appendage (LAA) is prepared for insertion of the index finger. A purse-string suture is placed over left ventricular apex (LV).

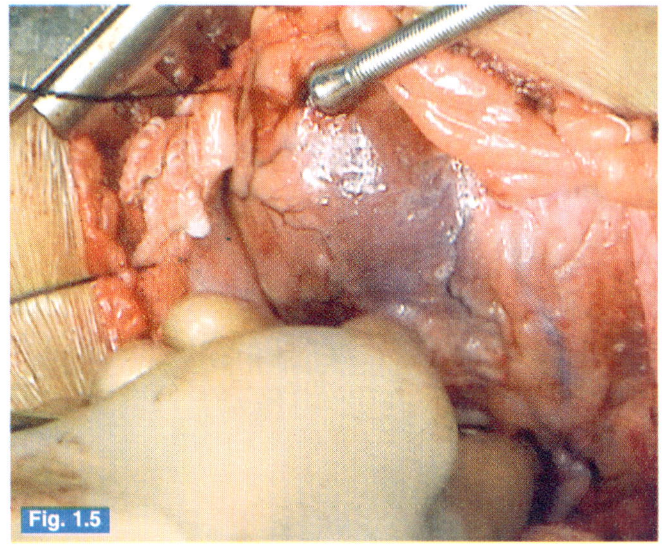

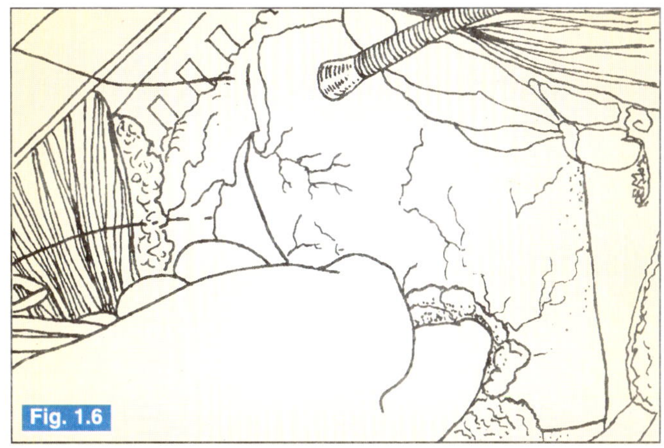

Figs 1.5, 1.6: Closed mitral valvotomy. The surgeon's right index finger is inserted through left atrial appendage.

A small (or large) sponge is placed on the diaphragmatic surface inside the pericardial cavity to elevate the left ventricular apex. An avascular area is identified and a 2-0 braided suture is taken in a horizontal mattress fashion. It is threaded through Roummel tourniquet. A small (2–3 mm) incision is made in the epicardium within the suture. The blunt end of the knife is used to enter the ventricular cavity and dilate the incision. The assistant then tightens the tourniquet to avoid blood loss.

The left atrial appendage is washed carefully and all clots and debris are removed. The surgeon inspects the Tubb's dilator and sets it to open to about 2.0–2.5 cm. He should ensure that on releasing the dilator it closes completely. The surgeon then washes his right hand and especially the right index finger. He then inserts the tip of the index finger in the left atrial appendage incision and holds the stay sutures in his right hand (Figs 1.5, 1.6). He removes the atrial clamp with his left hand while insinuating the index finger into the left atrial appendage avoiding any blood loss (some surgeons use a purse-string suture on a tourniquet to avoid bleeding).

The surgeon palpates the mitral valve apparatus, the mitral orifice and assesses the following: (a) pliability, (b) orifice size, (c) nodularity, (d) calcification, and (e) mitral regurgitation. He will then hold the Tubb's dilator in his left hand and insert the same through the apical incision directing it towards his right index finger in the mitral orifice (Figs 1.7, 1.8). Once the dilator tip is felt by the right index finger, it is pushed through the mitral orifice. The left hand is then used for gently opening the Tubb's dilator in the mitral orifice, while keeping it in contact with the index finger in the left atrium.

The surgeon can feel the valve open by a (give) feeling on the dilator. The dilator is then closed and the screw is adjusted to the desired final opening. Dilatation is repeated and the dilator is withdrawn into the ventricle. The index finger now palpates the

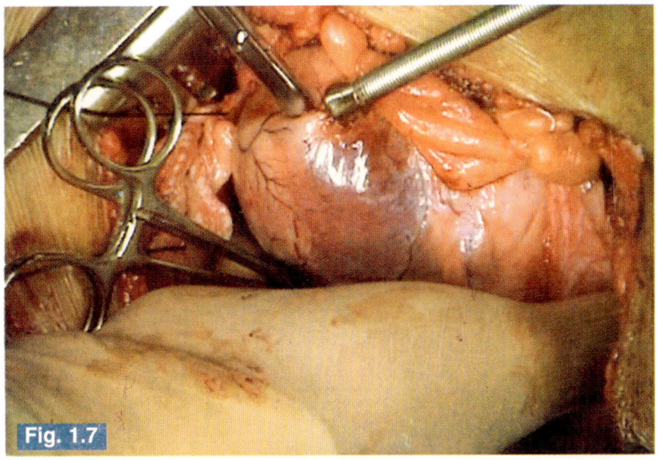

Fig. 1.7

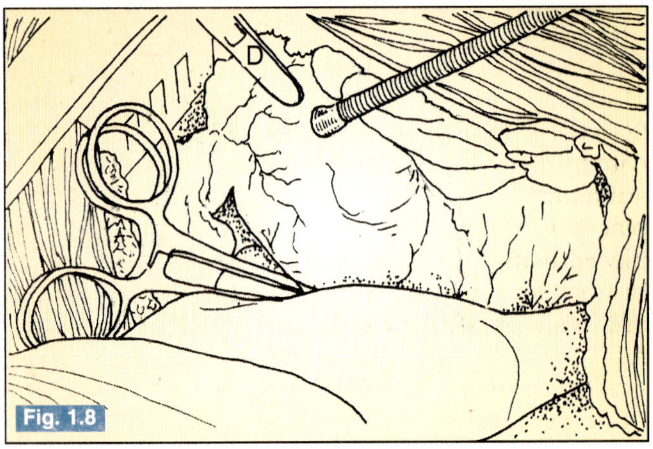

Fig. 1.8

Figs 1.7, 1.8: Closed mitral valvotomy. The surgeon's right index finger is inserted through left atrial appendage and Tubb's dilator (D) through left ventricular apical incision.

mitral valve for the result. It is sometimes possible (with experience) to mobilise the subvalvular fusion with the finger, once the dilator is withdrawn. If found satisfactory, the dilator is withdrawn from the heart while tightening the tourniquet. The commissures of the mitral valve should be open and the index finger is only withdrawn when the dilatation is considered adequate.

A 4-0 mattress suture is then used to approximate the left ventricular incision. Some surgeons prefer to tie down the 2-0 purse-string suture as well. The sponge behind the left ventricle is now removed.

The atrial appendage anterior to the incision is excised and a running 2-0 braided suture is used to close the left atrial appendage incision. A silk ligature is usually placed proximal to the atrial clamp as well for haemostasis. The pericardial cavity is washed and the pericardial incision is approximated with interrupted sutures. A 28–32 french drain is placed in the left pleural cavity through a separate incision and the wound is closed in layers.

Closed Mitral Valvotomy in Atrial Fibrillation

(also for Redo closed mitral valvotomy)

In patients with atrial fibrillation certain precautions are mandatory.

1. Stop oral anticoagulation at least 48 hr before surgery
2. Have one or two units of blood crossmatched and available in the operating room.

If the atrial appendage is small, contracted or feels boggy from a thrombus, the approach will be through the left atrial wall.

The left ventricular apex is prepared as before as a first step. The surgeon then places two concentric purse-string sutures of 2-0 braided suture at the junction of the left superior pulmonary vein and left atrium. The outer purse-string suture is held loosely in a Rummel tourniquet. A small haemostat is placed on the inner purse-string suture.

The surgeon washes the index finger of the right hand and prepares the Tubb's dilator. He will then make an incision inside the inner purse-string suture into the left atrium. The left hand index (or middle) finger is used to prevent bleeding. He will then dilate this incision with graduated Hegar dilators until an adequate size dilator is passed. He will then insert the right index finger or little finger and wiggle it gently to enter the left atrium and palpate the mitral valve. Dilatation is completed before attempting to withdraw the finger from the left atrium.

When dilatation is completed, the surgeon withdraws his finger while the assistant tightens the Rummel tourniquet. He will also apply gentle traction on the inner purse-string. The inner purse-string is tied first, followed by the outer purse-string. This is usually haemostatic.

The left ventricular apical incision is closed as described earlier. The pericardial cavity is washed and inspected for leaks.

It is very essential to palpate the femoral, dorsalis pedis and radial pulses in all extremities before transferring the patient to the intensive care unit. Rarely an embolectomy may be required if the pulse in any extremity is absent.

COMPLICATIONS

These include tear of the left atrial appendage, bleeding from the left ventricular incision, inability to dilate the mitral valve and severe mitral regurgitation. Occasionally there may be peripheral embolisation.

Bleeding from Left Atrial Appendage

In patients with normal sinus rhythm this is easily controlled by placing an occluding vascular clamp. Interrupted mattress sutures may be taken proximal to the clamp to ensure complete haemostasis. It is important to ensure that the surgeon does not panic in such a situation and takes necessary precautions to restore blood volume and obtain adequate haemostasis.

Apical left ventricular tears are best controlled with the finger. An appropriate sized Hegar dilator is the best instrument in such circumstances. Once the bleeding is controlled, sutures (pledgeted 4-0 polypropylene) can be placed to obtain satisfactory haemostasis.

If the mitral valve cannot be dilated or if there is severe mitral regurgitation then it is best to close the incision and return the patient to the intensive care unit. Transesophageal echocardiography can be performed to assess the need for urgent intervention. Only very rarely will immediate open heart surgery be required. In my experience of over 1500 closed mitral valvotomies, I have not had an occasion to convert to an open heart procedure on the table.

Femoral or brachial embolectomy will be necessary in the event of embolisation. It is best done before returning the patient to the intensive care unit.

RESULTS

Closed mitral valvotomy has been criticised as a blind procedure for a long time. However it cannot be denied that several thousand patients have had long term relief with this simple operation. It can be performed in hospitals not equipped for open heart procedures. It is inexpensive and can provide good immediate and long term relief. Operative mortality should be under 1% in patients with normal sinus rhythm and not more than 2% in patients with atrial fibrillation. The operation can (and has been) repeated safely in young patients with recurrent mitral stenosis.

OPEN MITRAL COMMISSUROTOMY / MITRAL VALVE REPAIR / MITRAL VALVE REPLACEMENT

Some general principles pertaining to the above procedures need elaboration. These are open heart procedures with direct vision intracardiac surgery. Before describing the actual procedure the reader should learn the surgical approaches to the heart, cannulation for cardiopulmonary bypass, and approaches to the mitral valve.

APPROACHES TO THE HEART

In the early development of open heart surgery midsternotomy was not popular. Once it became obvious that midsternotomy was possible and provided excellent exposure to all parts of the heart, it became the incision of choice. However, a right thoracotomy was used in early procedures for mitral valve surgery and has now become popular once again for cosmetic reasons. In addition, recently there is resurgence of a minimally invasive approaches for mitral valve surgery. A bilateral transverse thoracotomy (clam shell incision) is rarely used.

Right Thoracotomy

This procedure is recommended for patients under 20 years of age. This was a posterolateral thoracotomy in the past. It is now confined to a small submammary anterior thoracotomy. The patient is placed in a left semilateral position. A sand bag is placed behind the right scapula and one behind the buttock for support. The right leg remains extended and rests on a pillow placed over a flexed left thigh and leg. The right arm is placed over the patient's head with the forearm flexed at the elbow (Fig. 1.9). Skin preparation is from the chin to the groin including the right thigh up to its middle. The patient is draped leaving a window extending from the axilla to the subcostal region and from angle of scapula posteriorly to the left parasternal region. This provides an opportunity to change to a midsternotomy if needed. The right groin is draped and kept ready for femoral cannulation. This is a safety precaution and should not be overlooked.

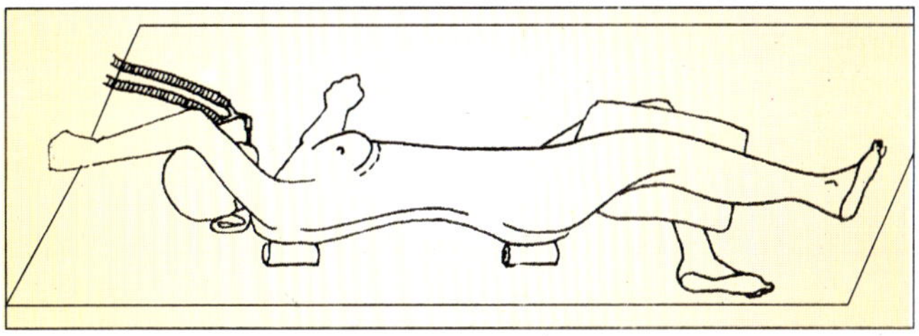

Fig. 1.9: Position of patient for right thoracotomy.

The incision is curved and semicircular. It follows the breast fold 1 cm away in young women and adolescents and is placed over the curve of the fifth intercostal space in men. Anteriorly it reaches the right border of the sternum and posteriorly does not extended beyond the midaxillary line (Fig. 1.10). The upper skin flap is grasped with Allis forceps and gentle dissection elevates the subcutaneous (breast) tissue to expose the fourth intercostal space. An

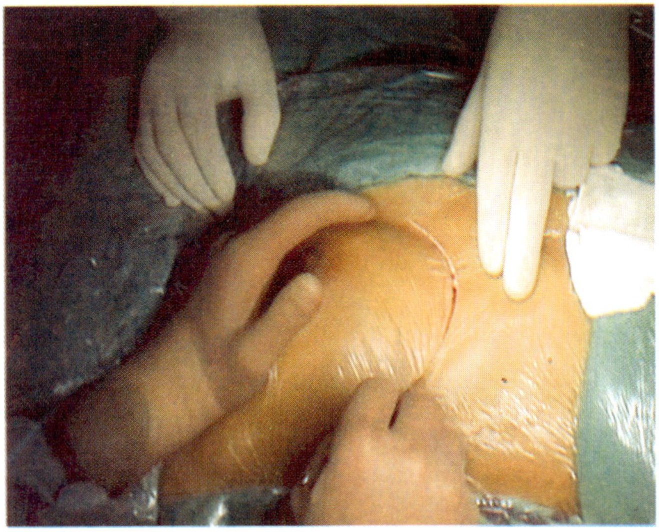

Fig. 1.10: Incision for right thoracotomy below and following the curve of the breast.

incision in the fourth intercostal space is made to enter the pleura. This incision is extended anteriorly taking care not to injure the right internal mammary artery. If it is divided, a 2-0 suture should be used to ligate both ends securely for haemostasis. Posteriorly the serratus anterior muscle is retracted and the intercostal incision is extended. A rib spreader (Burford, Harken retractor) is placed with the handle anteriorly and opened to provide adequate exposure. The right lung is retracted with a malleable retractor over a sponge. An incision 1 cm anterior and parallel to the right phrenic nerve is made in the pericardium (Figs 1.11, 1.12). The incision is extended downwards towards the diaphragm where it curves anteriorly. Superiorly, the thymus is dissected and retracted. The pericardial incision extends over the ascending aorta up to the reflection of the pericardium. The placement of stay sutures in the pericardium is important for adequate exposure (Figs 1.13, 1.14). Two sutures (2-0 braided) are placed in the pericardium at the highest point of reflection over the aorta. When pulled up, these will bring up the aorta forwards to the incision. Stay sutures are also placed (4-6 in number) on the right edge of the pericardium and pulled up strongly and fixed to the drape. This manoeuvre usually provides excellent exposure of the right atrium the superior and inferior vena cava and left atrium. When the right atrial appendage is retracted caudally the entire ascending aorta up to the pericardial reflection comes into view (Figs 1.15, 1.16). A simple purse-string suture is placed on the right atrial appendage and this is retracted caudally and held by an assistant (or a haemostat). Now it becomes easy to place a purse-string suture for aortic cannulation and also for the cardioplegia line. The patient can be

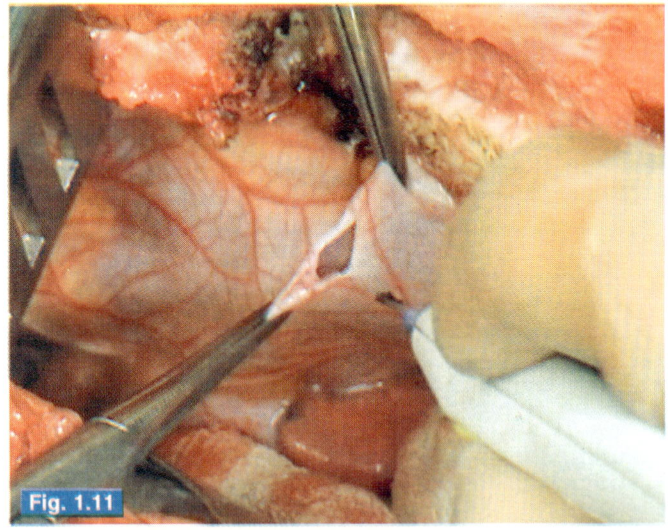

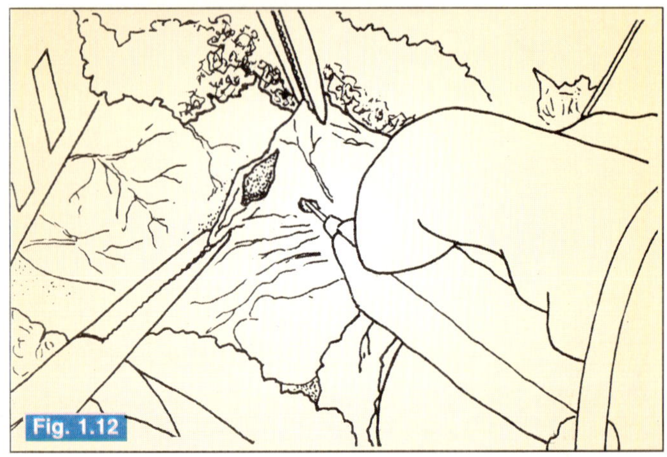

Figs 1.11, 1.12: The pericardial incision through right thoracotomy.

heparinised at this stage and purse-string suture may be placed over the inferior vena cava–right atrium junction.

Cannulation

The inferior vena cava is cannulated first followed by the superior vena cava. The superior vena cava purse-string is retracted by an assistant (or a haemostat). The adventitia of the aorta is grasped by a right angle clamp and held under downward traction by an assistant. To cannulate the ascending aorta an incision is made inside the purse-string sutures. The cannula is held in the right hand with the index finger occluding the opening — no clamp is placed on the cannula. If the cannula is a soft one, it is placed in ice cold saline for a few minutes before inserting. When the cannula is inside the aorta, the assistant clamps it with his right hand. In this way cannulation at a depth is accomplished without blood loss. In over 300 cases no complications were encountered during aortic cannulation

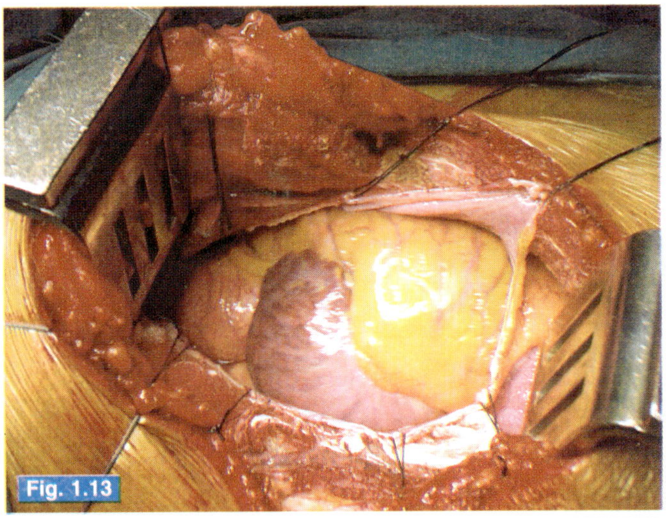

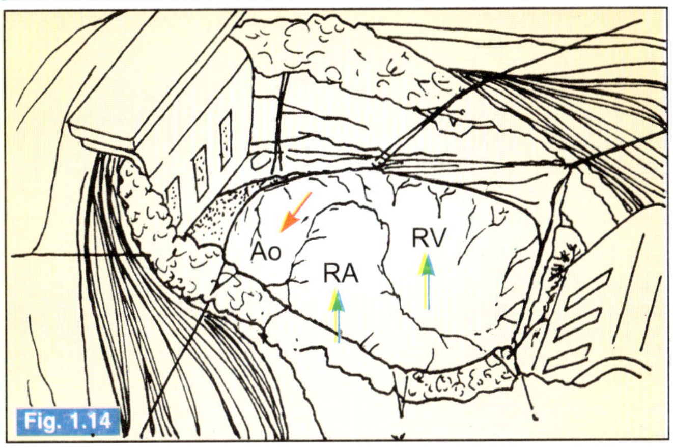

Figs 1.13, 1.14: Exposure of the heart through right thoracotomy. Aorta (Ao), right atrium (RA), right ventricle (RV).

and femoral cannulation was not required in any patient. Hegar dilators of appropriate size may be used to dilate the incision for cannulation.

The aortic purse-string sutures are used to pull up the aortic cannula and a silk suture is used to fix the cannula to the subcutaneous tissue. Cardiopulmonary bypass is now begun. The superior vena cava cannula is advanced into the superior vena cava and the purse-string suture on the right atrial appendage is retracted towards the foot end of the patient and held by the assistant (or a haemostat). The cardioplegia cannula is now inserted into the ascending aorta through a purse-string suture in its highest point of the curve leaving sufficient length of aorta for cross clamping. The cross clamp is now placed on the ascending aorta with the handle towards the foot end of the patient (Fig. 1.16a). In this way the cannulae and the cross clamp lie completely to the left of the incision giving free and unobstructed access to the aorta, right and left atria. The left atrium can now be incised behind the Waterston groove to decompress the left heart before infusing the cardioplegic solution into the aortic

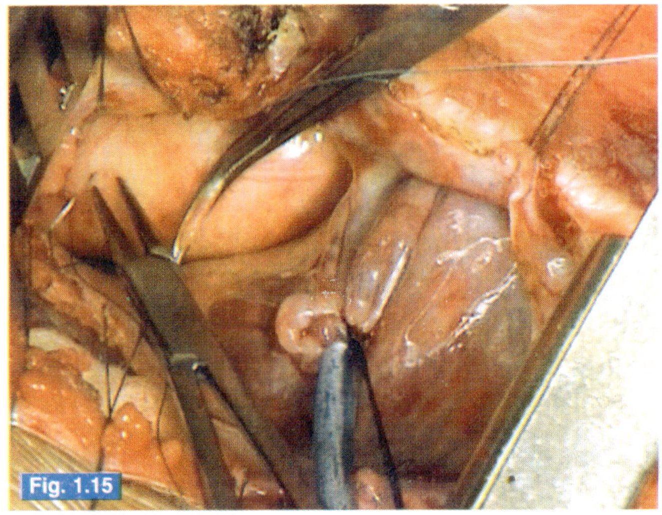

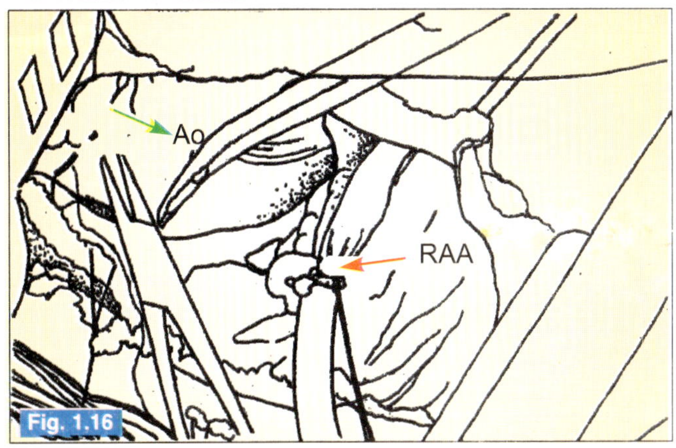

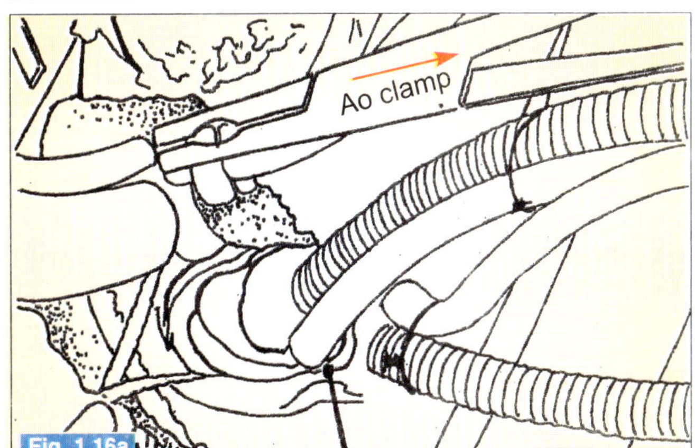

Figs 1.15, 1.16, 1.16a: Exposure of aorta through a right thoracotomy incision. Note site of aortic cannulation and retracted right atrial appendage (RAA), placement of aortic (Ao) clamp; arrow shows foot-end of patient in Fig. 1.16a.

root. All atrial septal defects, isolated ventricular septal defects (perimembranous or inlet type with correct preoperative diagnosis), mitral valve surgery (repair/replacement/redo mitral valve surgery) tricuspid valve surgery and aortic valve replacement can all be performed with ease through this incision. Occasionally a supracardiac variety of total anomalous pulmonary venous connection can also be corrected through this incision.

Once the surgery is completed, it is necessary to emphasise a few technical points. Placing a ventricular epicardial wire on the anterior surface of the right ventricle may pose a problem. However, the pacing wire can be easily placed on the diaphragmatic surface of the right ventricle over an avascular area. Both the atrial and ventricular wires are brought to the surface through the incision itself instead of through separate punctures. One of the reasons for re-exploration for bleeding in the author's experience was the point at which these wires penetrated the chest wall. When these wires were brought through the incision there were no bleeding complications.

Patients, specially young women, are delighted with the cosmetic result. With experience, the incision gets smaller in length and more invisible in the breast fold.

Standard Midsternotomy

This is the most widely used incision for all cardiac surgical procedures. It provides safety and adequate exposure to all parts of the heart and proximal great vessels, lungs, pericardium, etc.

The patient is placed in the supine position, with small pillow or a ring to support the head which is turned to one side (usually the left) for convenience. The left arm may be extended and supported on an arm rest. It can also be tucked by the side of the patient if necessary. Skin preparation is from the chin to the umbilicus. In patients undergoing a repeat median sternotomy the right groin is also prepared for emergency femoral cannulation. Drapes are placed to provide access from suprasternal notch to below the xiphoid process with sufficient exposure for placing drainage tubes. The right (or left) groin is also draped if necessary.

The Incision

Most surgeons begin the incision above the sternal notch and extend to 1–2 cm below the xiphoid. Such a long incision is generally required in elderly patients or in patients undergoing reoperation following a closed mitral valvotomy or previous sternotomy. In young patients the tissues are resilient and a more cosmetically acceptable skin incision can be used. This may begin 2–3 cm below the sternal notch and stop at the sternal xiphoid junction. We have used a 7–7.5 cm incision centred over the third intercostal space for cosmetic purposes with no difficulty for valve surgery. The knife is used to deepen the incision down to the periosteum of the sternum. A retractor is placed in the upper end of the incision and with blunt and sharp dissection the suprasternal notch is defined. Troublesome venous bleeding may sometimes be encountered at this time. A small sponge is packed into this area for a few minutes, it will then become easy to see and secure haemostasis. The retrosternal space is gently opened using a right-angled clamp and the soft tissue is divided with a cutting cautery tip down to the bone. The inter-clavicular ligament needs to be divided carefully, failing which the sternal saw may sometimes get stuck. The periosteal incision is carried down along the midline up to and beyond the xiphoid to the anterior rectus sheath. Haemostasis at this point will be required and all bleeding points from the periosteum need coagulation. There is always a constant vein anterior to the junction between the sternum and xiphoid. This will need careful coagulation. The sternal saw is now used to divide the sternum from above downwards (or below upwards) according to convenience. The sternal saw is applied to the sternum and the sternum is elevated at the same time when the saw is activated and drawn downwards (or upwards). At this time the lungs are completely deflated by the anaesthetist. This will avoid any injury to the pericardium and the cardiac chambers. Once the sternum is split a sponge is placed between and behind the two blades and haemostasis is secured. A sternal retractor is placed and the incision opened to expose the pericardium.

Interlocking Sternotomy

The incision on the sternum is curved in a lazy S shape. This provides a firmer fit and greater surface area for healing. It eliminates vertical slipping of the sternum and reduces postoperative pain. Care must be taken to keep the incision to the lateral confines of the sternum (Fig. 1.17). In more than a thousand such sternotomies performed by the author and residents there have been no complications.

Redo Sternotomy

In valvular surgery reoperations are quite common and one must be prepared for them. Sternotomy following a previous thoracotomy (right or left) is quite safe and poses no great risk of haemorrhage. However, a repeat sternotomy can be hazardous unless certain essential precautions are taken. The sternal split is done with the oscillating saw (Fig. 1.18). It is best to begin at the xiphoid. A mastoid retractor is placed on the skin and retracted to expose

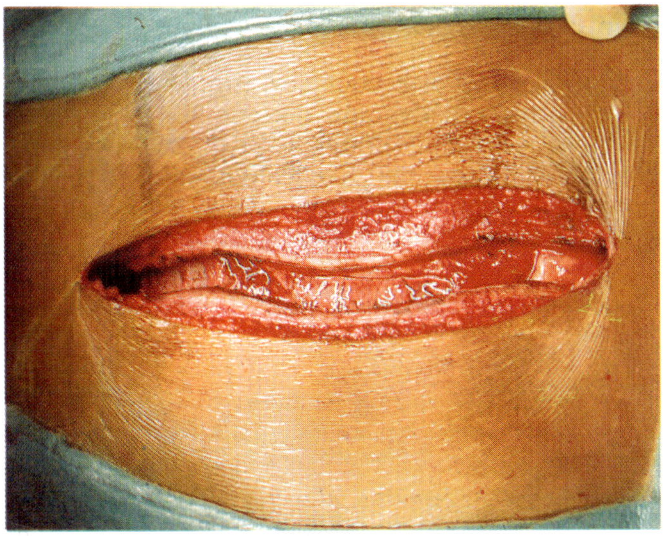

Fig. 1.17: Interlocking sternotomy.

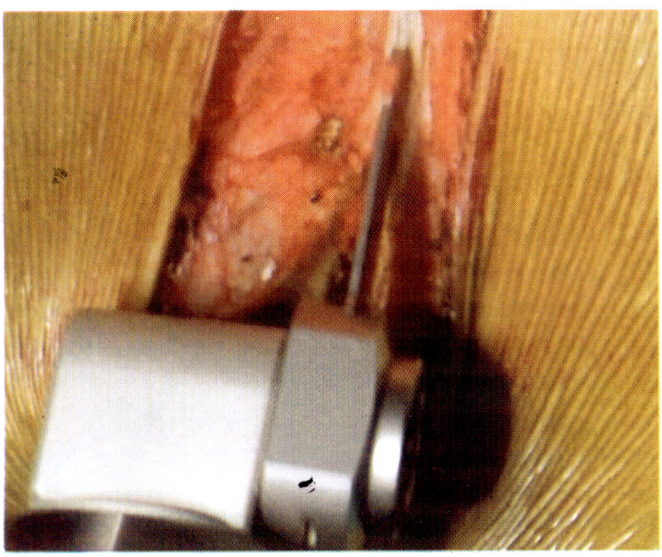

Fig. 1.18: Use of oscillating saw.

the xiphoid. The xiphoid is divided with heavy curved (Mayo) scissors.

Following this, dissection behind the xiphoid separates the heart from the xiphisternum. Using a blunt guaze tipped instrument (a Kelly forceps with a piece of gauze) gentle dissection behind the xiphoid and lower sternal end will provide sufficient safety to begin the sternal split. With the blade of the oscillating saw at an angle to the sternal surface the anterior table is split for about 1 to 2 cm from the xiphoid incision. At this point the saw is withdrawn. The mastoid retractor is advanced in a cephalad direction and opened to widen the split in the lower end of the sternal body. Using a nontooth tissue forceps, a piece of gauze is gently packed into the split and pushed behind the sternum as far as it will go, and left in place. The saw is now used to extend the sternal incision by a few centimetres by dividing the anterior table and carefully dividing the posterior table until the gauze is seen. The mastoid retractor may now be changed to a small (paediatric) sternal retractor which is pushed between the split lower end of the sternum and opened gently. This will allow further dissection to be carried out in the same manner as described above for a few more centimetres. In this way the entire sternum up to the suprasternal notch can be split safely with patience and care. It is necessary at this point to emphasise that great care must be taken at the manubrium-sternal junction and just above where the aorta or the innominate vein may be adherent to the posterior table of the sternum. This is most likely if the thymic tissue and pericardium are not closed at the first operation. This is also the point of greatest danger if the patient has had sternal infection or if the surgeon has used Teflon pledgets to close the aortotomy at the first operation and has failed to close the pericardium over the aorta.

In the author's experience of more than 300 redo sternotomy incisions there was one instance of aortic injury necessitating femoral cannulation and decompression of the heart to obtain adequate exposure. Some surgeons routinely use femoral cannulation and the ususal method of sternotomy on cardiopulmonary bypass for safety. However, it must be emphasised here that all cardiac surgery (especially open heart surgery) at present is palliative and necessitates reoperation, especially in patients under the age of 50 years. Therefore, it is very essential to take necessary precautions at the first operation (primary surgery) to avoid catastrophic haemorrhage at the subsequent operations, simply by approximating the pericardium (or thymus/ pleura) over the heart. The author has performed three and even four sternotomies in the same patient safely and without mishap.

Dissection of the Heart

Once the sternum is split, dissection of the heart is not difficult to accomplish. Two right-angled retractors are placed under the left blade of the sternum and held elevated by the assistant. Adhesions between the heart and the posterior aspect of the sternum can now be completely and carefully divided under vision with a cutting cautery tip. The surgeon may need to change position with the assistant to accomplish complete exposure of the heart on the right side as well. Patience, perseverance and care are necessary to avoid injuring the heart and great vessels. Once sufficient exposure is obtained, a sternal retractor is placed and opened wide. Dissection of the heart can now proceed safely within the pericardial sac under direct vision.

The heart may also be dissected free of adhesions on cardiopulmonary bypass. This may be necessary when the patient's haemodynamics are unstable, or if there is troublesome bleeding. This is especially required in patients with high right atrial pressure (tricuspid stenosis/tricuspid stenosis + tricuspid regurgitation) where decompression of the heart provides for safe dissection. Inevitably this will prolong the cardiopulmonary bypass time.

For safe and satisfactory mitral valve surgery the heart should be completely free within the pericardial sac. This may be quite natural in the large majority of first operations. However, in young patients with recent rheumatic activity and in patients with previous cardiac surgery, pericardial adhesions need to be carefully and completely divided to obtain complete exposure of the heart.

Pericardial adhesions in recent rheumatic activity are seen with an intact pericardium. In these patients it is best to open the pericardium between haemostats over the ascending aorta. The edges can now be held in haemostats and dissection can proceed with care using both blunt and sharp dissection. Rheumatic adhesions are fibrinous and generally yield easily on blunt dissection. Care must be taken to avoid arrhythmias which can be quite bothersome in some seriously ill patients. It is best to expose the aorta and right atrium, and decompress the heart on cardiopulmonary bypass and then complete the dissection in such patients.

In patients undergoing mitral valve surgery following a previous thoracotomy the pericardium on the anterior surface of the heart is intact. Again it is best opened over the ascending aorta to identify a plane of dissection and then extend the incision caudally. The left edge of the pericardium is then elevated by an assistant while the surgeon gently depresses the heart while dividing the fibrous adhesions with sharp dissection. Over the right ventricle. The dissection must meticulously adhere to the glistening undersurface of the pericardium, failing which the dissection may go too deep and separate epicardial coronary vessels (especially left anterior descending) from the heart with fatal consequences. All dissection is done under direct vision using blunt tipped metzenbaum scissors. When difficulty is encountered in one area it is best to proceed to another area where the plane of dissection is more clear. In this way with patience and care the heart can be separated from the pericardium.

In patients with congestive heart failure, pulmonary hypertension or severe cardiomegaly dissection of the left ventricular posterior and diaphragmatic surfaces is sometimes best performed on cardiopulmonary bypass with a decompressed collapsed heart.

In patients undergoing a repeat sternotomy where the pericardium has not been closed it will be necessary to carefully find the retracted edge of the pericardium. This will be seen on the right atrium on the right side and over the pulmonary artery or right ventricle on the left. Once these edges are seen they are held in haemostats and then the heart is dissected free within the pericardium. Occasionally bleeding or dense adhesions may preclude dissection of the heart from the pericardium. The left pleura can then be opened widely so that the heart falls into the pleural cavity. This facilitates exposure of the mitral valve, although it may pose problems in deairing and in ensuring satisfactory myocardial protection and topical cooling which are advantages of dissection of the heart.

Cannulation

Through the midsternotomy incision cannulation is performed in the usual manner with (a) ascending aortic cannulation at its highest point within the pericardium; (b) superior vena cava cannulation through the right atrial appendage; (c) inferior vena cava cannulation through the body of/at right atrium–inferior vena cava junction and cannulation just distal to the aortic sinus for cardioplegia. The superior vena cava and inferior vena cava are taped and retained in snuggers in patients with an atrial septal defect, or if tricuspid valve repair is required or anticipated.

In the right thoracotomy incision the inferior vena cava is cannulated first and the superior vena cava next. A silk ligature on the right atrial appendage at the cannulation site is used to retract the right atrial appendage towards the diaphragm exposing the ascending aorta. Aortic cannulation is made safe and easy by the following manoeuvres. Stay sutures are placed at the pericardial reflection from the aorta and pulled up to the drapes. The adventitia within the aortic purse-string sutures are divided and spread with the scissors. A right-angled clamp holds the adventitia of the ascending aorta and is retracted downwards and outwards by the assistant. The assistant holds a tube clamp in his right hand. The aortic cannula tip is placed in sterile ice slush to make it stiff. The surgeon holds the adventitial flap over the aortic purse-string with the tissue forceps in his left hand. An incision is made in the aorta with a No. 11 blade. The adventitial flap prevents bleeding from the aortotomy. The surgeon holds the aortic cannula in his right hand with the right index finger occluding it. It is then inserted into the ascending aorta and immediately clamped by the assistant. The surgeon then tightens the aortic purse-string sutures and fixes the cannula to the purse-string sutures with a silk tie. The cannula is now deaired and connected to the arterial line of the extracorporeal circulation. The cannula is fixed to the subcutaneous tissue with a silk suture. Cardiopulmonary bypass is begun by declamping the venous line and superior vena cava cannula. While the patient is still ejecting, the cardioplegia cannula is placed in the ascending aorta. The inferior vena cava cannula is now opened to venous drainage. Normothermic perfusion is preferred.

With a Minimal Sternotomy Incision

There is no difficulty in cannulating the aorta and the superior vena cava through the right atrial appendage. The inferior vena cava cannulation is usually done on cardiopulmonary bypass. The inferior vena cava right atrium junction (comes into view only when the heart is decompressed. The inferior vena cava cannula is connected to the Y on the venous line and clamped. A separate stab incision is made in the skin below the xiphoid. The inferior vena cava cannula is passed through this incision into the pericardial sac and then inserted through a purse-string suture into the inferior vena cava. This skin incision can later be used for placing the pericardial drainage tube. In this way even through a small skin incision mitral valve surgery can be performed with ease.

EXPOSURE OF THE MITRAL VALVE

Through a Midsternotomy Incision

In Patients with Atrial Septal Defect + Mitral Valve Disease

After clamping the aorta, antegrade cardioplegia is completed and the superior vena cava and inferior vena cava tapes are snugged, tight. The right atrium is opened from right atrial appendage towards the inferior vena cava cannulation site (watch for air in the venous line). Two stay sutures of 4-0 braided silk on the anterior lip of the incision are pulled up and clipped to the drapes. Two additional stay sutures on the transverse muscle band (linea terminalis) are tied to the pericardium. This provides excellent exposure of the right atrium without an assistant's help.

A Mayo retractor is now placed on the edge of the septal defect and retracted by the assistant. If the septal defect is small it may be extended by an incision towards the inferior vena cava. The mitral valve now comes into view. Correction of mitral stenosis/mitral regurgitation can now be performed under direct vision. A 4-0 braided suture can also be used on the edge of the septal defect to retract the atrial septal defect for better exposure.

In Patients who have a Small Left Atrium

The incision is the same, behind the right interatrial groove. If the approach is through a right thoracotomy, the exposure of the mitral valve is excellent. If through a sternotomy, then some manoeuvres may be required for good exposure. These are: (1) Complete mobilization of the heart inside the pericardium, all adhesions must be divided; (2) separate superior vena cava/inferior vena cava cannula; (3) left atrial incision extends into oblique sinus behind the inferior vena cava; and (4) table is rotated to the left for about 10°–15°. With these manoeuvres it is quite easy to get good exposure of the mitral valve (Figs 1.19, 1.20). In over 4000 mitral valve surgeries the author has not failed to obtain adequate exposure for successful surgery.

Transeptal Approach

Some surgeons believe that an extended transeptal incision provides better exposure in a small left atrium.

The right atrial incision is made in a transverse direction from the right atrium to the space between the two right pulmonary veins. With both the right atrium and left atrium open the septum is incised across the fossa ovalis. Stay sutures separate the two septal halves providing adequate exposure of the mitral valve.

A Superior Transeptal Approach

Here the incision in the left atrium is at first made in the Waterston groove. It is then extended across to the roof of the left atrium behind the superior vena cava. This incision may sacrifice the sinoatrial nodal artery with the possibility of postoperative atrial arrythmias. A Cooley retractor can now be placed in the left atrium for exposure of the mitral valve. If this is still not satisfactory the superior vena cava/inferior vena cava tapes are snugged and the atrial septum is incised from the lateral to the medial (septal cusp) direction.

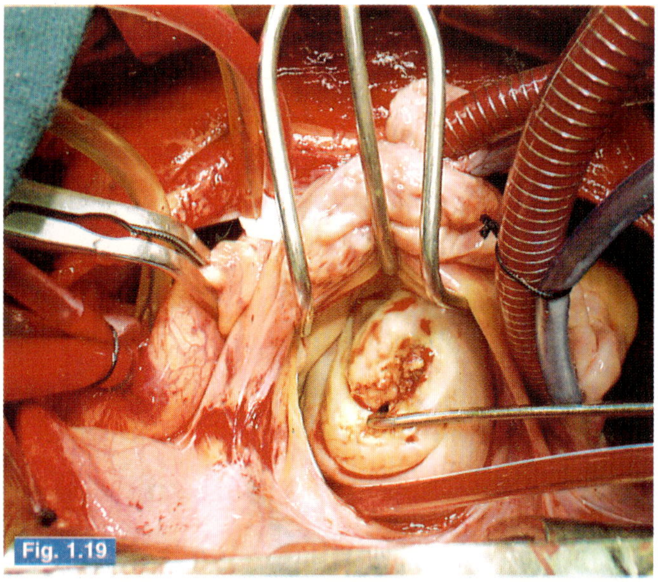
Fig. 1.19

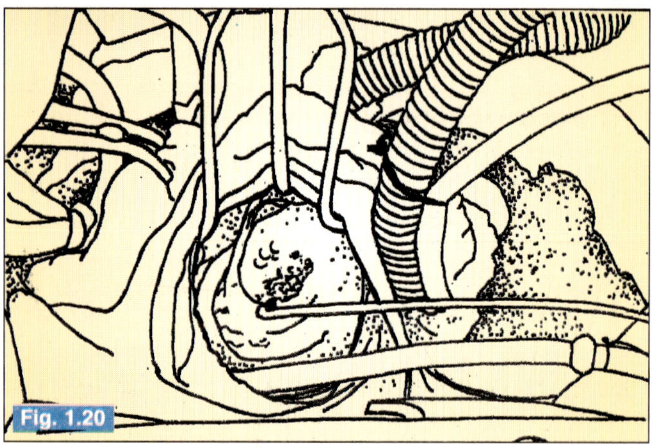
Fig. 1.20

Figs 1.19, 1.20: Exposure of mitral valve through a standard left atrial incision.

Another Approach to the Mitral Valve

In patients undergoing both aortic and mitral valve surgery, sometimes it is possible to perform the mitral valve replacement through the aorta. This is done without incising the right atrium/left atrium. Generally the aortic root diameter in such patients exceeds 30 mm. This approach was popularised by Denton Cooley and later demonstrated by Stanley Crawford. The aorta is opened widely with an oblique or transverse incision. Three stay sutures are placed at the commissures of the aortic valve and pulled up to the drapes. The aortic leaflets are excised and all calcium and fibrous material is carefully excised and the left ventricle thoroughly washed. The anterior mitral leaflet can now be detached completely exposing the mitral orifice (Figs 1.21, 1.22). After decalcification an appropriate sized mitral valve can be sewn with continuous or interrupted sutures. It must be emphasised that the orientation of the mitral valve must be correct and prechecked before taking the first stitch. Failing to take this precaution may place a mitral valve in the reverse position with serious consequences. After the mitral valve has been seated the aortic valve may be replaced in the usual manner.

Caution: In this approach a small left atrial or left atrial appendage thrombus can easily be missed. The surgeon must take adequate steps to inspect thoroughly both the left atrium and left atrial appendage before seating the valve. Deairing is then performed through the aorta.

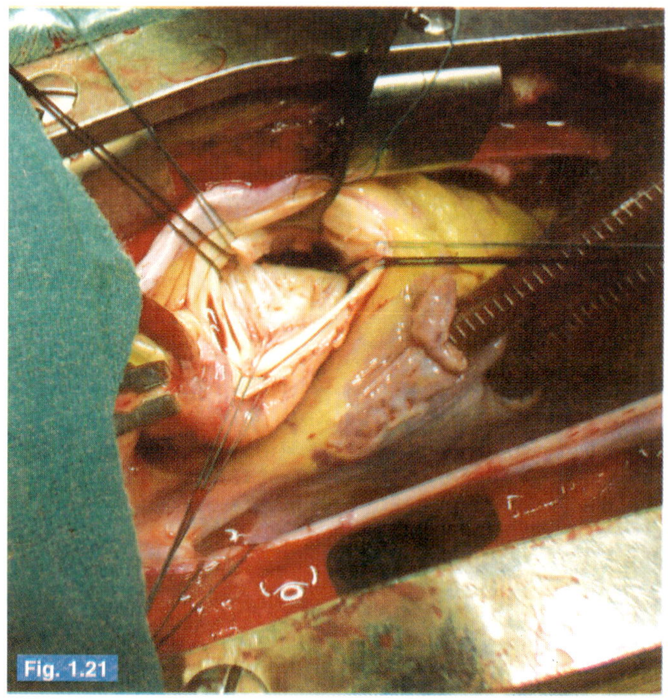
Fig. 1.21

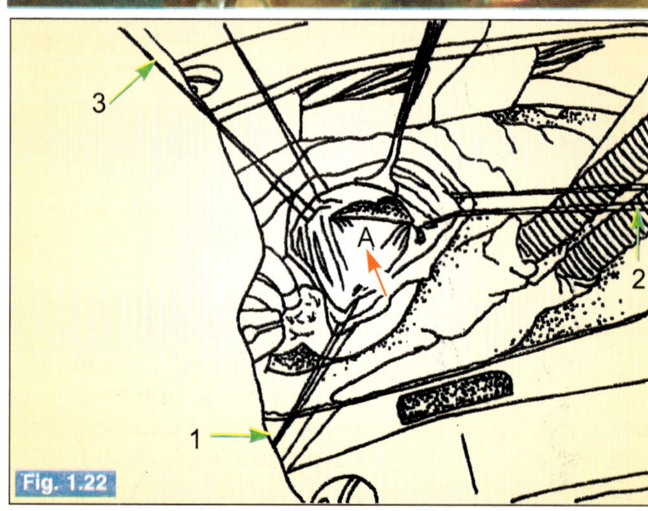

Fig. 1.22

Figs 1.21, 1.22: Exposure of mitral valve through aorta. Note stay sutures 1, 2 and 3 through aortic commissures and anterior mitral leaflet (A).

Other Approaches

Other uncommon approaches rarely used include a superior approach (Fig. 1.23). In a large dilated left atrium, the roof is accessible between the aorta and superior vena cava. The exposure of the mitral valve through this approach is excellent.

Another approach is to transect the aorta transversely well above the commissural pillars. The divided aorta is retracted anteriorly exposing the entire roof of the left atrium. This approach can be used in patients who require both aortic and mitral valve surgery.

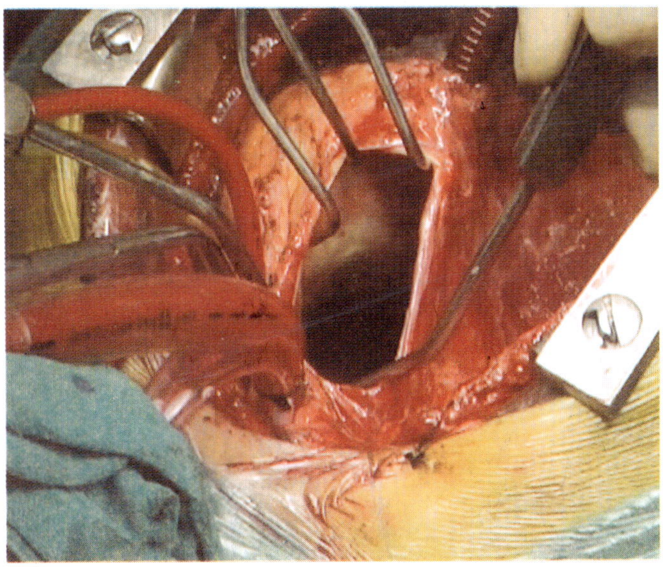

Fig. 1.23: Exposure of the mitral valve through the roof of left atrium.

Mitral Valve Surgery through the Left Ventricle

Although this may not sound convincing, the author has had an opportunity to replace the mitral valve through the left ventricle. This is quite likely to happen in a patient with a large inferior wall aneurysm with severe mitral regurgitation. When the left ventricular cavity is open one can visualise the scarred and contracted posterior papillary muscle. This observation precludes the possibility of repairing the mitral valve. In this situation again the mitral valve can be replaced through the incision in the left ventricle. Once again it is essential to ensure proper orientation of the mitral valve, in order to avoid any mishaps. Once the mitral valve replacement is completed the left ventricular incision can be closed and the left ventricular cavity can be deaired before tying the final suture. The exposure of the mitral valve through the left ventricle is one of the best providing the surgeon a full view of the entire mitral valve apparatus and the left ventricular outflow tract.

These are approaches to the diseased mitral valve. The surgeon is the best judge in any individual case to decide which approach and what technique he will use for any particular patient. Some of these techniques will provide considerable time saving during surgery and may be adapted with advantage.

OPEN MITRAL COMMISSUROTOMY

Indications

The indications for open mitral commissurotomy include the following:

(a) Mitral restenosis (following a previous closed mitral valvotomy or mitral valve balloon dilatation).

(b) Mitral stenosis with atrial fibrillation and a left atrial (or appendage) thrombus.

(c) Mitral stenosis with aortic stenosis or aortic regurgitation, or organic tricuspid valve disease (tricuspid stenosis or tricuspid regurgitation).

(d) Mitral stenosis with an atrial septal defect "Lutembacher's syndrome".

(e) Mitral stenosis with minor degree of calcification in a young patient.

Preoperative Assessment

Must include a transoesophageal echocardiography intraoperatively. This examination is best performed by the surgeon himself. The following need careful assessment.

(a) Spontaneous echocontrast in the left atrium suggestive of severe mitral stenosis.

(b) Left atrium or left atrial appendage thrombus.

(c) Thickness and mobility of anterior mitral leaflet and posterior mitral leaflet.

(d) Subvalvular fusion and calcification.

(e) Mitral regurgitation, if any.

Instrumentation

To perform a satisfactory valvotomy, the surgeon will need the following instruments.

(a) A Cooley (or Carpentier) mitral valve retractor.

(b) A pair of long-handled steel hooks.

(c) A good long handled No. 11 knife.

(d) A fine right-angled clamp.

(e) A Debakey right-angled vascular clamp.

(f) A pair of Russian tissue forceps and a pair or two of Debakey vascular forceps.

(g) A 16 or 14 F (Bard or Sarns) left atrial vent.

Technique

As soon as the cardioplegic solution is delivered antegrade the left atrial incision is widened superiorly behind the superior vena cava and inferiorly behind the inferior vena cava. A Cooley retractor (or a Carpentier self-retaining retractor) is placed and the atrial septum is retracted anteriorly and to the left by an assistant. A vent is placed with its tip in the left inferior pulmonary vein and put on negative suction providing a clean and dry field. The atrial cavity is carefully cleared of any organised and fresh thrombus ensuring that the atrial appendage is completely inverted. If the thrombus is large or long-standing and organised it can be peeled off the left atrial wall by blunt and sharp dissection almost like an endarterectomy. Once the thrombus and all debris are meticulously cleared the left atrial cavity is washed several times over with cold saline to ensure complete removal of all debris.

The mitral orifice is inspected. A curved hook is placed, one under the posterior cusp and one under the anterior mitral leaflet and retracted. This usually puts in relief the line of fusion (Figs 1.24, 1.25). With a No. 11 blade an incision is made in the commissure close to the annulus. A right-angled clamp is introduced through this incision and directed towards the mitral orifice. The commissure is now incised under vision with the No. 11 knife, from the annulus towards the orifice. This separates the anterior mitral leaflet and posterior mitral leaflet at the anterior commissure. Using the similar technique the posterior commissure is also incised. The subvalvular apparatus now comes into full view and can be easily separated by the hooks. Using the No. 11 blade and a pair of long Pott's scissors the subvalvular fusion is separated and the incision in the papillary muscles is carried down to the base assuring clear and complete separation of the papillary muscle into anterior and posterior portions. This is repeated at the other commissure as well. At this stage fusion of the chordal apparatus from the tip of anterior mitral leaflet to the tip papillary muscles will be in clear view of the surgeon.

Cusp Thinning

The next step is to remove all the excess fibrous tissue deposited on the anterior mitral leaflet and posterior mitral leaflet. The surgeon grasps the anterior mitral leaflet firmly with a Russian forceps. Using a Debakey tissue forceps, the fibrous peel is separated at the annulus and pulled in a downward direction towards the mitral orifice (Figs 1.26, 1.27). This fibrous peel is grasped in a right-angled forceps and excised carefully with a No. 11 knife at the free edge of the anterior mitral leaflet. A similar procedure on the posterior mitral leaflet will separate the fibrous peel that imprisons the posterior mitral leaflet.

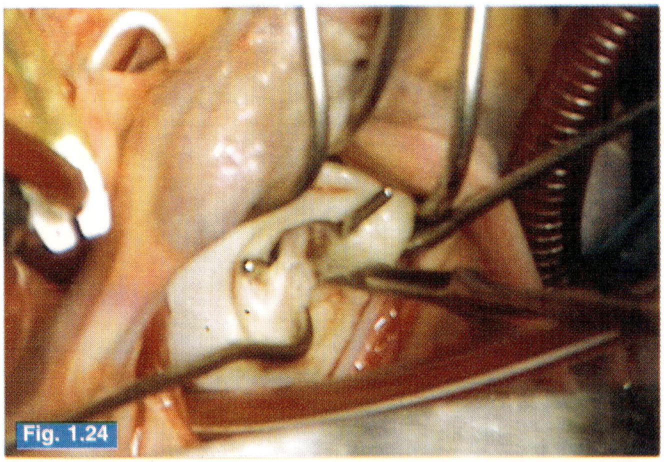

Fig. 1.24

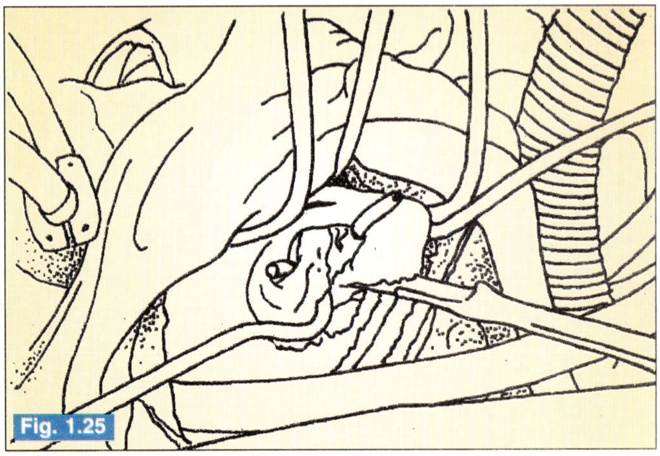

Fig. 1.25

Figs 1.24, 1.25: Technique of open commissurotomy, the separation of subvalvular fusion.

Fenestration

The Debakey vascular right-angled forceps is now applied to the tip of the papillary muscle at the anterior commissure. Without crushing, the subvalvular fusion is brought into view. The surgeon grasps the fibrous tissue with a vascular forceps in the left hand and this is separated by blunt and sharp dissection until the chordae are clearly visible. If it fails to come off with ease, an incision is made into the fused chordal apparatus removing a wedge of fibrous tissue between the anterior mitral leaflet and papillary muscle tip. A similar procedure is performed at the anterior and posterior papillary muscle heads on both sides.

Assessment

When the procedure has been completed it is necessary to check if the cusps move freely, if the

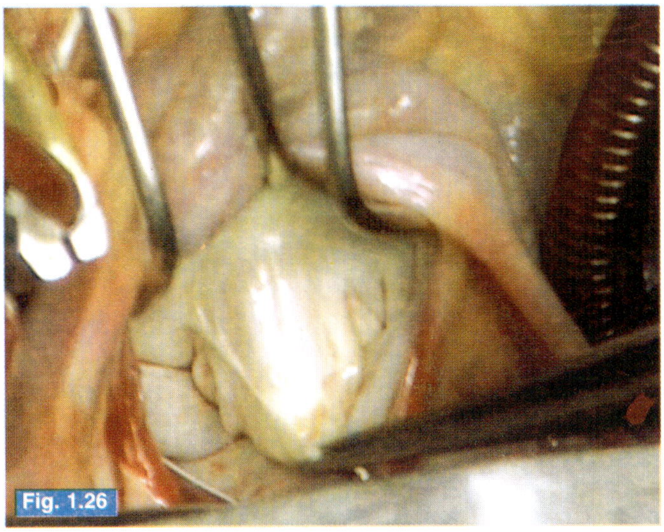

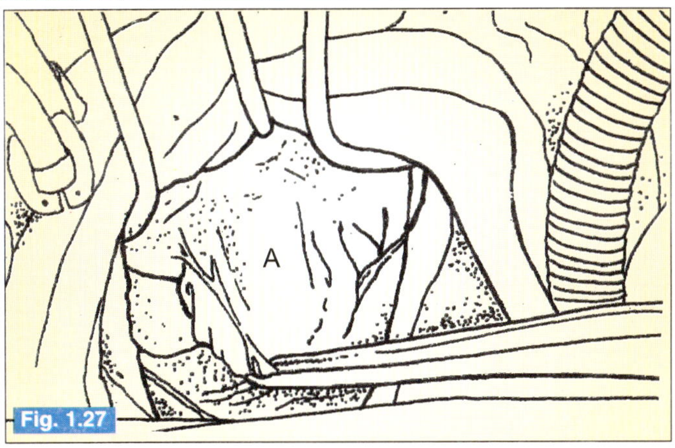

Figs 1.26, 1.27: Technique of cusp thinning. Note the glistening surface of anterior mitral leaflet (A).

mitral opening is full and if there is any mitral regurgitation. By using a bulb syringe filled with saline all of the above can be checked by injection 50–75 ml of saline through the mitral valve. If the cusps are mobile they will be seen to float up and coapt with each other. Spaces along the commissure will be the points at which mitral regurgitation Jets can be visualised. Generally, the commissural ends are the points at which mitral regurgitation is always (almost always) found following commissurotomy. It is generally necessary to do a commissuroplasty to ensure competence. This can be accomplished at both ends. Briefly a double-armed 4-0 polypropylene suture is used. The needles are passed about 3–4 mm away from the point of leak (mitral regurgitation) from the ventricular aspect on the annulus towards the atrial aspect. The posterior needle is now passed through the free edge of the posterior leaflet (where it is thick and firm) and back again through the annulus. When this suture is tightened and tied the annulus is reduced by about 4–5 mm and the posterior leaflet is tucked under the anterior mitral leaflet at the commissure. This usually restores competence. A similar suture is placed at the other commissure as well. Sometimes mitral regurgitation jets are also found at the junction of the scallops of the posterior mitral leaflet. This is especially so in rheumatic heart disease where the cusps are retracted. A double-armed 5-0 prolene mattress suture restores competence at such points.

After placing these sutures the valve is again tested by injecting saline with a bulb syringe into the left ventricle. Care must be taken to keep the aortic vent line (cardioplegia line) open so that all air gets expelled instead of being pushed into the coronary arteries. If the valve is found competent then air and saline will be expelled through the aortic line instead of leaking back through the valve.

At this stage the surgeon must decide if the correction is satisfactory. Minor jets of mitral regurgitation can be accepted. However, if the cusps are stiff, immobile or not coapting sufficiently for competence, it is best to replace the valve.

Before proceeding further it is safe to invert the left atrial appendage into the left atrial cavity and inspect for hidden fresh or organised thrombus. It must be removed with meticulous care and the atrial appendage and cavity washed thoroughly with strong suction (to be discarded) to ensure that tiny pieces which may have fallen into the left pulmonary veins are aspirated. The anaesthesiologist may ventilate the lungs to assist in this step.

Deairing

A 28 F or 32 F chest drainage tube is then inserted into the left ventricle with the last sidehole positioned in the left atrium. This tube is held in this position by a suture to fix it to the pericardium. The left atrial incision is closed around this tube. At this stage the surgeon may want to release the aortic clamp and rewarm the patient. There is no danger of air embolism at this stage. Once the atrial incision is closed a mattress suture is placed loosely around the tube and held in a haemostat for later use. When the heart resumes satisfactory contractions the anaesthesiologist is asked to ventilate the lungs vigorously to evacuate air from the pulmonary veins The venous return line is partially clamped and the perfusionist warned to watch the level. The patient's head is elevated about 10° to 15°. The surgeon places his right hand around the heart using index finger to invert the left atrial appendage and massage the left pulmonary veins. The thumb is used to massage the right pulmonary veins. After adequate massage the hand is withdrawn and the chest retractor is held firmly and the patient chest is rocked vigorously while blood level remains above the left atrial suture line inside the pericardium. The anaesthetist now holds the lungs in inspiration. The blood pool level in the pericardium is maintained well above the left atrial suture line. The tube is withdrawn while the purse-string suture is held taut or tied by the assistant. The aortic vent line is placed on strong negative suction (300 ml/min). The heart will begin ejections soon. The blood in the pericardium is retrieved by the cardiotomy suckers. The clamp on the venous line is removed. With the heart empty and beating, the left atrial suture lie is reinforced, and inspected for leaks. The left atrial appendage is best ligated with a silk suture at this stage. The heart can now be defibrillated to sinus rhythm if necessary.

The patient can now be weaned from cardiopulmonary bypass. The aortic vent line remains on strong suction for at least 5 min. The aortic perfusion line is inspected for air bubbles which usually show up once cardiopulmonary bypass is discontinued. This may have to be removed before transfusing blood from oxygenator. A transoesophageal echo may now be performed to assess the mitral valve function. If the result is satisfactory (no mitral stenosis and no more than trivial to mild mitral regurgitation) the heparin may be reversed with protamine. If the result is unsatisfactory (moderate to severe mitral stenosis/ mitral regurgitation) cardiopulmonary bypass is resumed and proceed to replace the mitral valve.

Results

Open mitral commissurotomy is a standard procedure and provides excellent early and midterm results in young patients. Late results are dependent on age at operation. Under 35 years of age there is a greater risk of reoperation due to recurrent rheumatic activity. This risk increases with decreasing age despite prophylaxis with penicillin. In patients over the age of 35 years one can expect a good long term result. The greatest advantage is the normal or near normal haemodynamic correction and avoidance of anticoagulants. Operative mortality does not generally exceed 2% for uncomplicated patients.

MITRAL VALVE REPAIR

(Reconstruction)

Mitral valve repair is indicated in symptomatic patients with mitral regurgitation, with or without additional mitral stenosis.

Aetiology of combined mitral regurgitation and mitral stenosis is always rheumatic. However, pure mitral regurgitation may be as follows.

1. *Congenital:* Cleft mitral valve, atrial septal defect and mitral regurgitation or other valvular abnormalities.
2. *Rheumatic:* The large majority of patients have rheumatic heart disease in most developing countries. Pure mitral regurgitation in rheumatic heart disease is usually due to annular dilatation.
3. *Degenerative:* Myxomatous degeneration of the mitral valve is the most common cause of mitral regurgitation in developed countries. In India it accounts for about 5% of all patients with mitral regurgitation. It causes prolapse of either the anterior mitral leaflet or posterior mitral leaflet with ruptured chordae at times.
4. *Ischaemic:* Ischaemic mitral regurgitation is usually seen in less than 5% of all patients with mitral regurgitation. In this condition the mitral valve apparatus is almost normal except for the papillary muscle or ventricular wall. Repair is usually the operation of choice.
5. *Infective:* Infective endocarditis may cause severe mitral regurgitation by rupture of chordae or perforation of cusps. It is usually seen in patients with preexisting mitral or aortic valve disease. In patients with aortic valve disease the mitral valve may be quite normal in morphology before becoming infected.
6. *Post operative:* Iatrogenic mitral regurgitation is sometimes seen following balloon dilatation, closed mitral valvotomy or open mitral commissurotomy. Usually these valves are so deformed that repair is rarely possible.

Surgery

Before making a decision the surgeon must review the available information. It is best to avoid a repair in patient with a calcific valve and those returning for reoperation following failed repair or open mitral commissurotomy.

An intraoperative transoesophageal echocardiography is mandatory for assessment of repairability and to assess results of repair. It is important for the surgeon to learn this simple technique in order to assess repairability. Observation of the various parts of the mitral valve apparatus in its dynamic functioning state provides an excellent insight to the surgeon who will then visualise, in the arrested open heart, the exact cause. This will help him also to perform a satisfactory repair.

Technique

There are several techniques used for mitral valve repair. However all of them have the same basic principles. These include proper assessment, understanding of the cause and restoration of competence. They all use some method of reducing or remodelling the annulus especially in the posterior two-thirds to obtain proper coaptation of the cusps. The steps of operation are as follows.

(a) Establishment of cardiopulmonary bypass.

(b) Exposure of the mitral valve.

(c) Assessment.

(d) Correction of abnormality.

(e) Reassessment of valve function.

(f) Deairing.

(g) Closure.

(a) Cardiopulmonary bypass: This is established as described before. Briefly bicaval and ascending aortic cannulation and antegrade aortic root infusion of cardioplegia are used. Approach to the heart may be by a standard midsternotomy incision or by a submammary right thoracotomy incision. A minimally invasive approach via a right parasternal incision may also be used but is not described here.

(b) Exposure of the mitral valve: In patients with an enlarged left atrium (as in chronic mitral regurgitation) the best approach is via an incision just behind and parallel to the right interatrial groove (waterston groove). A generous incision 5–6 cm in the left atrial wall provides excellent exposure of the entire mitral valve apparatus.

Other approaches may be used in small left atria as in patients with acute mitral regurgitation and ischaemic mitral regurgitation (see approaches).

A Cooley retractor is placed in the left atrium to retract the septum and provide exposure of the mitral valve apparatus. In patients undergoing reoperation it will be necessary to mobilise the entire heart by dividing the pericardial adhesions for a satisfactory exposure of the mitral valve apparatus. Before attempting to assess the mitral valve any fresh or organised thrombus is first removed from the left atrium / appendage.

(c) Assessment: For those beginning to attempt mitral valve repair this step may take considerable time. However with experience one can easily discern the abnormalities quickly and proceed. Visual inspection or the anterior mitral leaflet and posterior mitral leaflet for thickening, calcification, perforation and for abnormal clefts is made. Two hooks are passed under the anterior mitral leaflet and posterior mitral leaflet at the anterolateral commissure and the leaflets are retracted. This exposes the commissural area; fusion of cusps, chordae and papillary muscles is noted along with any calcification. The thickness and pliability of the cusps can also be easily assessed by this step. Similarly the posteromedial commissure is also exposed and inspected. The hook is then passed under the posterior mitral leaflet to assess pliability and fusion. Further assessment is possible only after commissurotomy in patients with significant mitral stenosis. In patients with pure mitral regurgitation further assessment is made by injection of cold saline with a bulb syringe into the left ventricle. This will show if mitral regurgitation is central, eccentric or, if there is prolapse due to chordal rupture or elongation. One must also look for and find endocardial thickening in the left atrium, the so called 'jet lesion' or McCallum's patch. Location of this patch gives a clue to the pathology and site of abnormality. It is found on the atrial aspect of the anterior mitral leaflet when the posterior mitral leaflet is prolapsing and behind the posterior mitral leaflet when the anterior mitral leaflet is prolapsing. It may also be seen on the atrial septum in posteromedial commissural prolapse and at the base of the left atrial appendage in anterolateral commissural prolapse. If one is present its location and size are noted and the leaflet that is prolapsing can then be located.

Correction of Prolapse

If the prolapse is due to chordal elongation, the technique to correct is chordal shortening. Two techniques have been used in clinical practice. Chordal shortening at the papillary muscle level (Carpentier technique) or at the cusp level. Cusp level chordal shortening is simpler to perform and provides predictable long term results (Figs 1.28, 1.29).

A 4-0 suture is passed through the tip of the papillary muscle whose chordae are elongated and need shortening. The suture is pulled up to the drapes. This will deliver the subvalvular apparatus into the mitral orifice. A 5-0 suture (prolene) is used to impale the chorda to be shortened at the appropriate level (Fig. 1.30), the other end of the 5-0 suture is passed through the free edge of the anterior mitral leaflet where the chorda is inserted (see illustrations). When the suture is tied the chorda will be shortened (Fig. 1.31). This can be repeated on other chordae as well. Up to six chordae may be shortened by this technique. On completion of the procedure the 4-0 stay suture on the papillary muscle

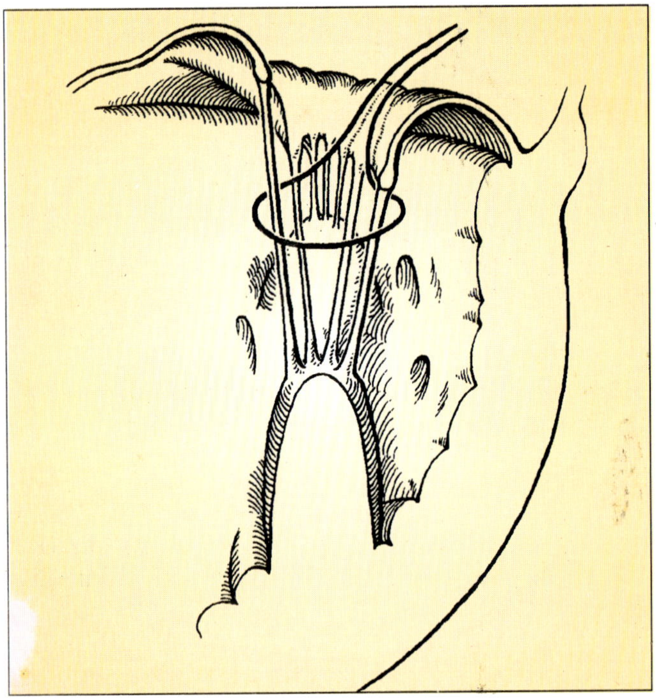

Fig. 1.28: Technique of chordal shortening. A silk suture is passed around both the chordae to be shortened and the opposite (posterior cusp) chorda.

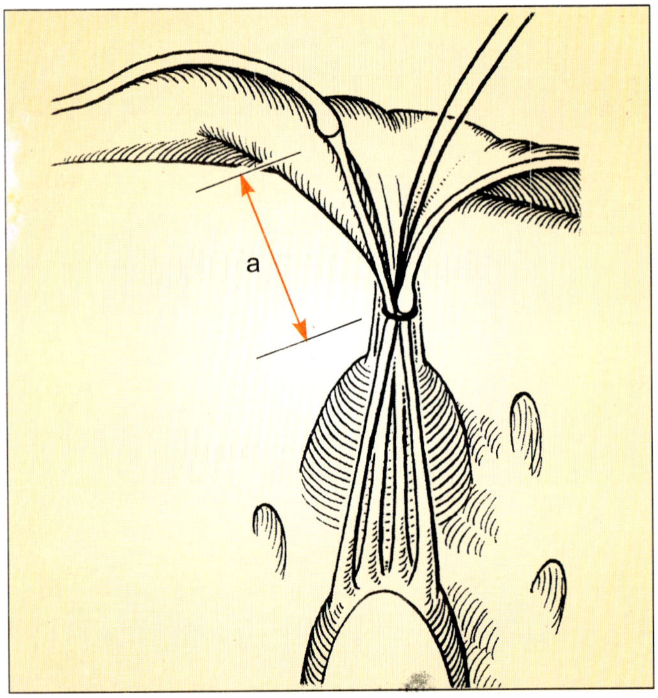

Fig. 1.29: After the left ventricle has been filled with saline solution, the silk suture is tightened so that the anterior mitral leaflet's degree of prolapse can be assessed and the length of chorda to be shortened (a) can be determined.

can be released. Injection of saline into the left ventricle will now demonstrate if the prolapse is adequately corrected.

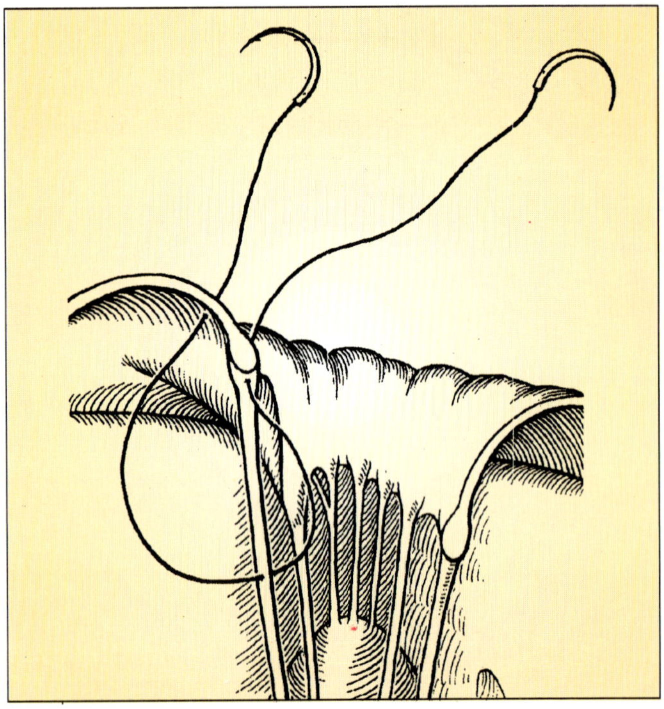

Fig. 1.30: After exposure of the chorda with a traction suture (not shown), a 5-0 polypropylene double-armed suture is taken, and the needle is passed through the chorda and then through the edge of the anterior mitral leaflet close to its point of attachment.

In the Carpentier technique the elongated chord or chordae are folded and buried in a trench created by incising the papillary muscle head. Adjustment of chordal length requires judgement in this technique.

Prolapse due to Ruptured Chordae

Chordal rupture due to infective endocarditis is the usual cause. The infected ruptured chorda is resected, especially if a vegetation is attached to it. The resultant prolapse is corrected by chordal transfer from the posterior mitral leaflet. An appropriate chorda from the posterior mitral leaflet arising from the same papillary muscle (anterolateral or posteromedial) is chosen. A 5-0 polypropylene sutured is used. Both needles are passed through the free edge of the posterior mitral leaflet where the chorda to be transferred is attached. While the assistant applies traction on this suture, a quadrangular portion of posterior mitral leaflet is cut away from it using a No. 11 blade. The needles of the suture are now passed through the free edge of the anterior mitral leaflet where the transferred chorda is to be attached. The suture is tied. The deficiency in the posterior mitral leaflet is closed with a 5-0 horizontal mattress suture. Injection of saline into the left ventricle will now demonstrate correction of prolapse.

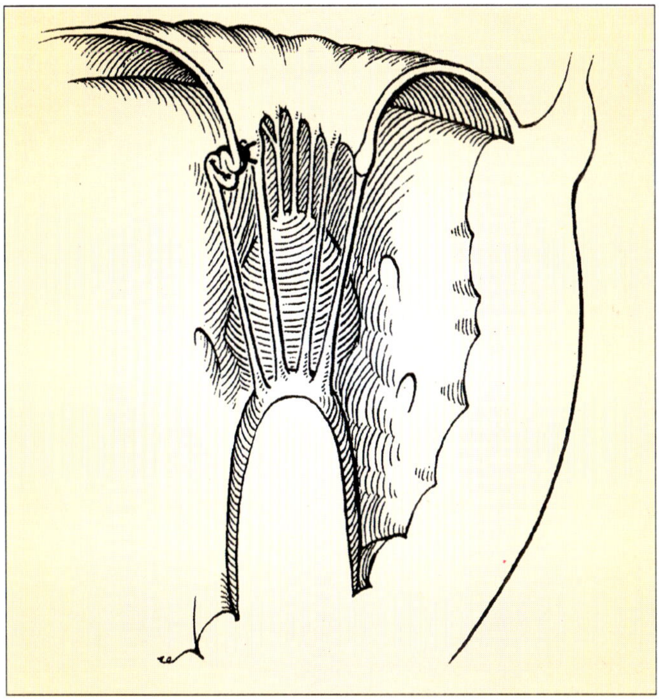

Fig. 1.31: The polypropylene suture is tied, shortening the chorda at cusp level. (Figs 1.28–1.31 reproduced with permission from *Texas Heart Institute Journal.*)

Myxomatous Prolapse

Prolapse may also result from rupture of chordae with myxomatous degeneration of the mitral valve. It usually affects the posterior mitral leaflet. In this case a quadrangular resection is the best technique for correction.

The prolapsing portion of the posterior mitral leaflet is identified by injecting saline into the left ventricle (Figs 1.32, 1.33). A 4-0 prolene suture is used to mark the edges of the prolapsing segment by passing each needle through either ends of the segment. A quadrangle of the posterior mitral leaflet from free edge to annulus is resected (Figs 1.34, 1.35). Another 4-0 prolene suture is used to close the gap in the annulus by a horizontal mattress suture. The cut ends of the posterior mitral leaflet are approximated with the previously placed 4-0 prolene suture (Figs 1.36, 1.37). Additional mattress sutures are used to obtain a firm and complete approximation of the edges of the posterior mitral leaflet. The valve is tested for competence by injecting saline into the left ventricle (Figs 1.38, 1.39).

If the prolapse affects the anterior mitral leaflet, a triangular segment of the anterior mitral leaflet is resected. The base of the triangle is at the free edge. It is better to resect less rather than too much. The cut ends are approximated with a 5-0 prolene horizontal mattress suture. Once again the correction is tested by injecting saline.

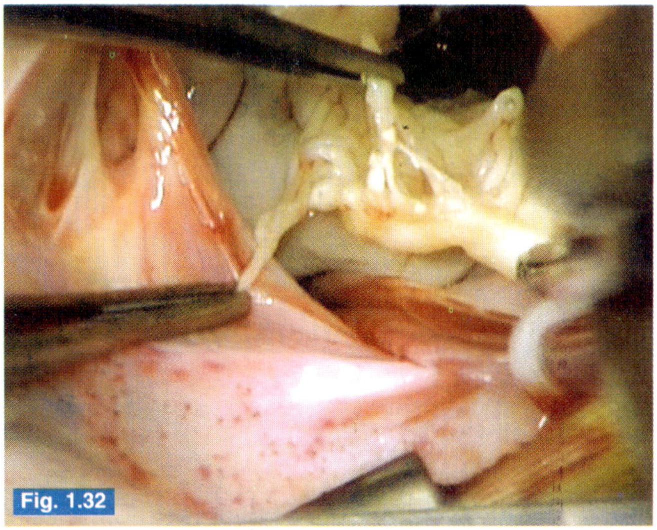

Fig. 1.32

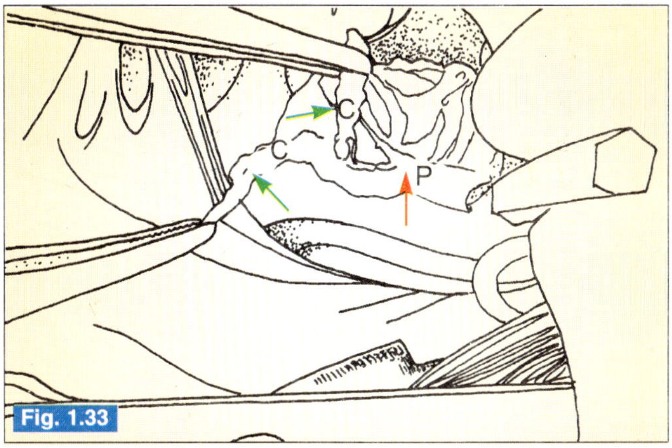

Fig. 1.33

Figs 1.32, 1.33: Myxomatous mitral valve. Note the ruptured chordae (C) and prolapsing segment of the posterior mitral leaflet (P).

Annuloplasty

Normally the line of closure of the mitral valve is well below the level of the annulus as seen in the 2 D echo (or transesophageal echocardiography). Dilatation of the annulus can be identified if the two cusps are seen to rise up to the level of the annulus during left ventricular systole. Such patients will benefit from annuloplasty.

Annuloplasty is also necessary to be performed when chordal shortening, transfer or quadrangular resection of the posterior mitral leaflet is performed. This is to support the chordae and leaflets and to reduce the tension on such repair procedures.

Several annuloplasty techniques have been described in the literature. However, the basic principle of all these is to reduce the posterior two-thirds of the mitral annulus (the attachment of posterior mitral leaflet) and to bring it forward for proper coaptation with the anterior mitral leaflet.

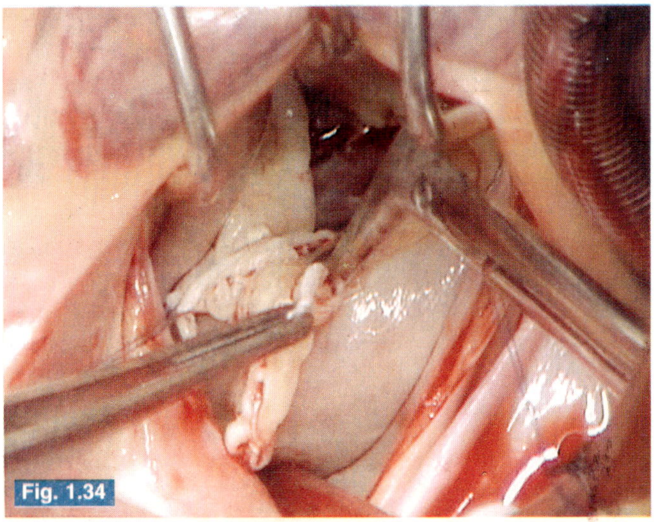

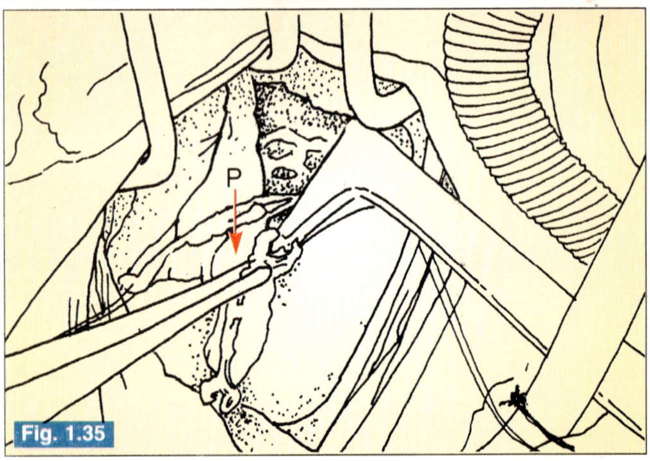

Figs 1.34, 1.35: Technique of quadrangular resection. The prolapsing portion of the posterior mitral leaflet (P) is resected.

This will also shift the line of coaptation between anterior mitral leaflet and posterior mitral leaflet to below the level of the mitral annulus as in the normal heart. In addition, this procedure will also increase the area of coaptation (contact) between anterior mitral leaflet and posterior mitral leaflet and abolish prolapse and mitral regurgitation.

The technique described here is a modification of the originally described technique of Denton Cooley. This technique is easy to learn and apply, is cost effective and provides good early and long term correction of mitral regurgitation. It is based on the principle of reducing the posterior annulus to fit it to the size of the anterior mitral leaflet. It is therefore essential to ascertain before hand whether the anterior mitral leaflet is pliable and mobile enough to provide a satisfactory final result.

Two silk sutures or two loops are passed through the anterior and posterior chordae of the anterior mitral leaflet. Gentle outward traction on these two silk sutures brings the anterior mitral leaflet into relief. The anterior mitral leaflet is measured using a regular valve sizers. The selected sizer is then placed on a piece of Teflon felt and marked. A C-shaped ring is cut out from it. The ends are trimmed. The ring is clipped by the centre to the drapes using a haemostat.

Generally nine sutures are required for this technique. Five green or blue sutures of 2-0 braided polyester (ethibond, 17 mm) are first placed as follows. The first suture is placed at about the 10 O'clock position (the centre of the anterior mitral leaflet is 12 O'clock) in a horizontal mattress fashion. This is the left trigonal suture. The trigone can be easily identified by gentle traction on the anterior mitral leaflet near the anterior commissure. Both needles are passed through the end of the C ring. The second suture is placed at the right fibrous trigone (2 O'clock position) and passed through the end of the C ring. The third suture is placed at the 6 O'clock position, a couple of millimetres behind the posterior annulus. The ends of this suture are passed through the centre of the C ring and held on a

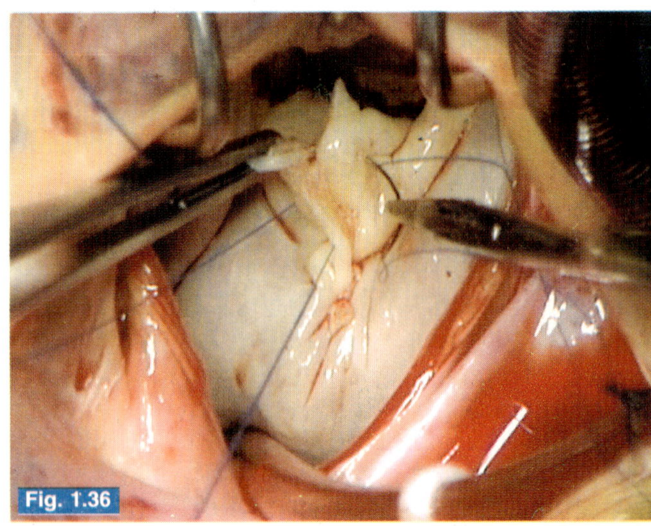

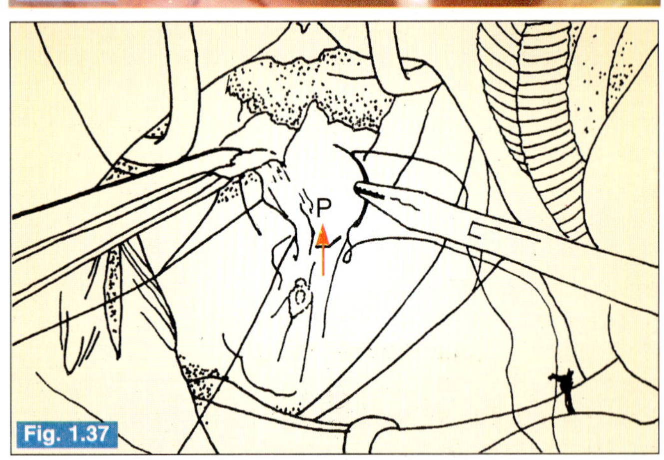

Figs 1.36, 1.37: Suturing the adjacent ends of the posterior mitral leaflet (P) after quadrangular resection.

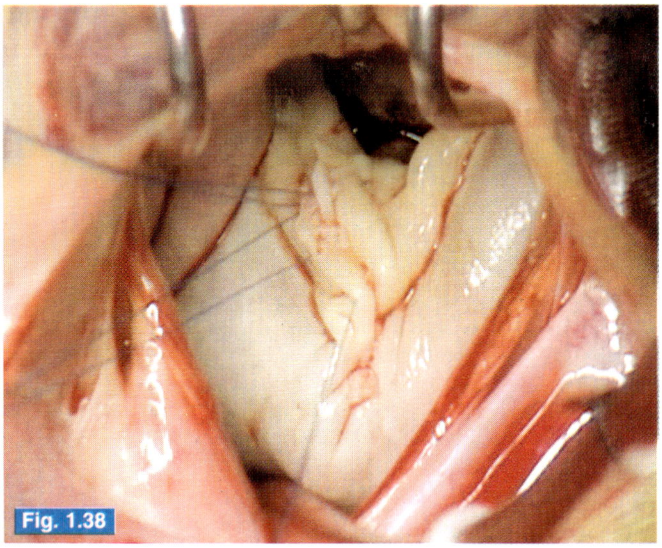

Fig. 1.38

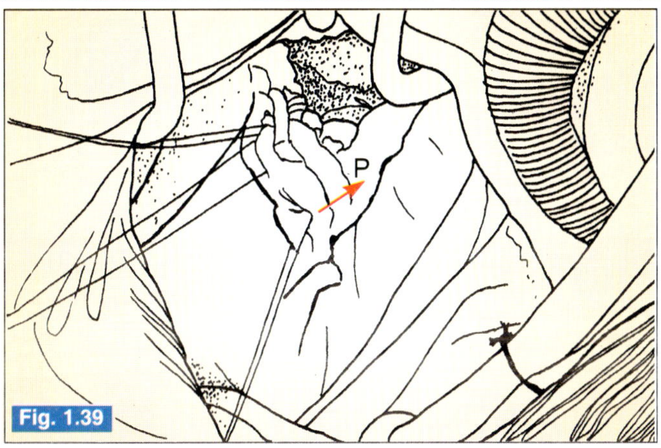

Fig. 1.39

Figs 1.38, 1.39: Completed quadrangular resection of the posterior mitral leaflet (P) using horizontal matters sutures.

haemostat. The fourth suture is placed on the posterior annulus about (8 O'clock in position) midway between the first and third sutures. These needles are passed through the Teflon ring at the appropriate position. The fifth and last (green) suture is placed midway between the second and third sutures about the 4 O'clock position, and the needles are passed through the Teflon felt ring.

Four white sutures (2-0 ethibond 17 mm) are now taken. The portion of the posterior annulus between the green sutures, at 9 O'clock, 7 O'clock on the left and 3 O'clock and 5 O'clock on the right are covered by these. These sutures are taken and both needles are now passed in the same sequence on the Teflon felt ring. All sutures are placed 2–3 mm behind the posterior annulus. These sutures should never be placed in the annulus. The Teflon felt ring is now lowered into the left atrium and the sutures are tied, in the same sequence as they were placed. Competence of the valve is tested by injecting saline. It is best to keep the aortic vent line open when injecting saline into the left ventricle on completion of the repair. This will avoid air being pushed into the coronary arteries if the mitral valve is competent. A semicircular fusion line between the anterior mitral leaflet and posterior mitral leaflet (the smile) [Figs 1.40, 1.41], transparency of the anterior mitral leaflet and displacement of the line of coaptation towards the left ventricle are indicators of successful correction of mitral regurgitation. Gentle all round pressure on the filled left ventricle will easily demonstrate any residual mitral regurgitation at this stage.

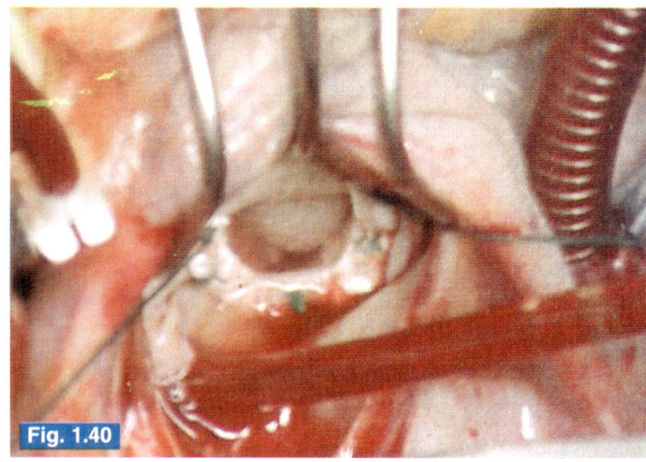

Fig. 1.40

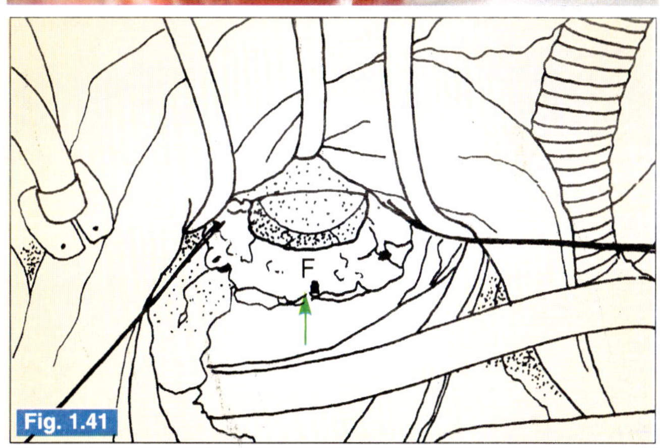

Fig. 1.41

Figs 1.40, 1.41: Completed posterior annuloplasty with a teflon (F) collar. Testing the mitral valve. Note the "Smile".

Cleft Sutures

In rheumatic heart disease fibrosis and contraction of the cusps produces acquired clefts between the scallops of the posterior mitral leaflet. Such clefts occasionally result in eccentric mitral regurgitation. These are best closed by a 5-0 horizontal mattress suture approximating the adjacent free edge of the posterior mitral leaflet scallops. One or two such clefts may require approximation in any patient.

When mitral valve competence has been seen to be satisfactory, one may proceed to close the left atrial incision.

Deairing

Following any type of repair, deairing the left heart chambers is extremely important. The heart must be allowed to beat while keeping the mitral valve incompetent and allowing air to be expelled from the left atrial suture line.

A soft 28 F (or 32 F) chest drainage tube is passed through the mitral valve into the left ventricle. The last sidehole of the tube is positioned in the left atrium. The tube is fixed to the pericardium using a suture and held on a haemostat. The left atrial incision is closed around the tube. A separate purse-string suture is placed around the tube on the left atrial incision. A blunt tissue forceps is placed in the left atrium to keep the left atrial incision open.

The aortic clamp is released with strong suction on the aortic root vent (cardioplegia line). This is done with the patient's head tilted down. The head end is now raised above the horizontal level so that intra-cardiac air gets sucked out of the aortic root vent which will be the highest point of the aortic outflow. The heart resumes beating, or may be defibrillated.

While the anaesthesiologist ventilates manually the venous drainage tube is partially clamped. With the right hand over the heart the index finger inverts the left atrial appendage and massages the left pulmonary veins towards the heart. The thumb of the right hand massages the right pulmonary veins in similar fashion. The other fingers of the right hand gently massage the left ventricle while the heart is beating.

While maintaining a blood level within the pericardial sac the sternal retractor is held in both hands and the heart is vigorously agitated inside the pericardial sac. One must ensure that the heart is beating vigorously and ejecting into the pericardiac sac through the open left atrium. When satisfied with the deairing the anaesthesiologist is asked to hold the bag in inspiration. With the heart immersed in blood the suture retaining the drainage tubes in the left atrium is divided. The forceps and tube are withdrawn. The purse-string suture is tied inside the blood level. The aortic vent is put on strong suction (300 ml/min). All residual blood in the pericardial cavity is sucked; the clamp on the venous line is removed. The heart should now be ejecting vigorously into the aorta. The patient is now weaned from cardiopulmonary bypass. With satisfactory haemodynamics (aortic and right heart pressures) and sinus rhythm (if possible), a transesophageal echocardiography is performed to assess the repair, if satisfactory heparin is reversed and the wound is closed in usual fashion.

Correction of Atrial Fibrillation

Although several procedures like the maze I, II, III, IV are described and new techniques such as electrocautery, radio frequency and cryoablation have been used, surgery for atrial fibrillation remains an individual surgeon's choice. In the author's experience simple direct current (DC) shock conversion on the table provides long-term (10 years) sinus rhythm in nearly 35% of patients. In addition, it preserves natural atrial transport function. It is successful in patients with a reasonable thickness (3–4 mm) of the left atrial wall. Patients with thin parchment-like atria, with near complete absence of muscle, are unlikely to revert to sinus rhythm.

The technique involves isolation of atrioventricular conduction pathways around the left valve (mitral) and around the pulmonary vein orifices. The endocardial lesions can be produced using a knife (classical Cox maze) a radio frequency probe or bipolar electrocautery. The operation extends cardiopulmonary bypass time by 20–30 minutes and is not free of complications. Ten-year results show 37–40% conversion and persistence of sinus rhythm and is not significantly different from simple synchronised direct current shock.

Results

Mitral valve repair is feasible in the large majority of cases and can provide good long-term results. The results are best in pure mitral regurgitation. However, in combined mitral stenosis and mitral regurgitation good results can be obtained in the large majority of patients with non calcific valves. Long-term (15–20 year) follow up has shown that nearly 30% of these patients may return for reoperation. This must be viewed in the light of the young age of these patients. Survival with mechanical valves is comparatively poor in these patients. Long-term survival (and therefore reoperation) is superior with valve repair. In addition, reoperations carry less risk in the current era, especially if the surgeon closes the pericardium.

MITRAL VALVE REPLACEMENT

Mitral valve replacement is indicated in patients with calcific mitral valve disease, mitral restenosis, failed mitral valve repair and in some patients with infective endocarditis, when repair is not feasible. In centres where surgeons are not trained in repair procedures, mitral valve replacement becomes the only choice.

Choice of Substitutes

Mechanical valves are the most commonly offered choice for the majority of patients. They are freely available in all sizes, and are suitable for all aetiologies, and are easy to implant. In addition almost all cardiac surgeons (experienced or not) have performed this operation during their training. Choice of mechanical valves is dependent on the surgeon or institution. However, in the author's experience no mechanical valve is superior. They are all obstructive, produce thromboembolic complications, require lifelong anticoagulation and are expensive. While the manufacturers claim superior haemodynamic performance, implanted valve function is dependent on several other factors. These include size of valve, method of implantation, orientation, *in situ* gradients, presence of infection, myocardial preservation, preservation of chordal apparatus and postoperative anticoagulation or antiplatelet medication.

In general mechanical valves are to be considered the best choice for young patients (under 35 years), for reoperations, for those who already have a mechanical valve in aortic position for inexperienced surgeons and on patient's demand.

Tissue Valves

Almost all bioprosthetic valves (tissue valves) currently in use for mitral valve replacement are stented. A stentless (Quatro) valve is still undergoing clinical trial but does not appear promising. Tissue valves are indicated in the elderly (over 40 years' age in India) and in patients who have contraindications for anticoagulant therapy. They may also be implanted in young women of child bearing age if the patient is willing to accept the risk of early degeneration and reoperation. One may choose from a variety of bioprostheses. However, the bovine pericardial valves appear to have a slight advantage in durability compared to the porcine aortic valves. They are all expensive and provide a 15–20 year reoperation free survival in the majority of patients.

The Pulmonary Autograft

This is to be considered in carefully selected patients. It is especially useful in uncorrectable congenital mitral valve lesions in infants and children. It is also recommended as the most suitable choice for patients over the age of 35 years. It is not recommended for patients with associated aortic or tricuspid valve disease or for reoperations.

This operation requires the availability a suitable homograft for right ventricular outflow tract reconstruction and should be performed by a surgeon with reasonable experience in mitral valve repair and replacement. The operation is complex, requiring skill and judgement and reasonable accuracy in assessment.

Surgical Technique

Excision of the Mitral Valve

Complete excision of the mitral valve is detrimental for good early and late results. The annuloventricular continuity must be maintained. The physiology of chordal preservation is explained in the accompanying figures.

Chordal Preservation

CW Lillehei demonstrated the importance of chordal preservation in mitral valve replacement as early as 1967. Subsequently several techniques have been developed and applied for chordal preservation. It is now clearly demonstrated that chordal preservation in mitral valve replacement offers vital advantages which include: (a) Preservation of left ventricle geometry and function; (b) reduction of early and late mortality; (c) improvement of late survival; and (d) prevention of ventricular rupture.

In addition, it is now clearly demonstrated that preservation of both anterior and posterior chordal apparatus alone provides the above advantages. Preservation of only posterior or only anterior chordae does not provide the patients with all these advantages. In the author's experience it is possible to preserve all chordal apparatus in 100% of patients undergoing mitral valve replacement. Of the various techniques described, Miki's technique is easy to learn, perform and does provide advantages over other techniques. It does not cause gradients in left ventricular outflow tract and permits implantation of a large valve.

The physiology of chordal function and the pathophysiology of chordal excision are explained in Figs 1.42, 1.43. Progressive dilatation and thinning of left ventricular muscle mass causes late left ventricular dysfunction and reduction of life span. Preservation of all chordae preserves ventricular size, geometry, function and improves late survival and function.

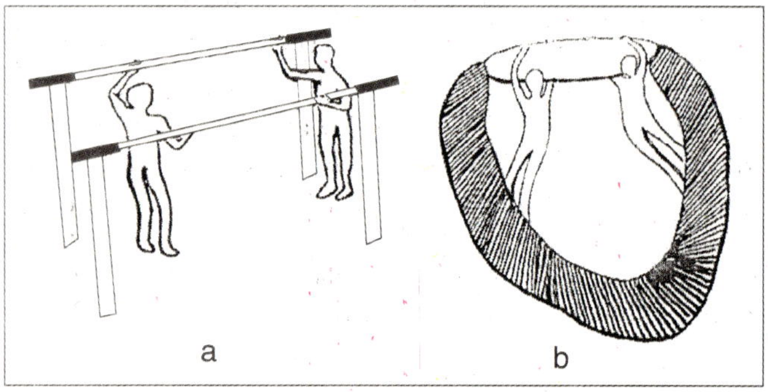

Fig. 1.42: The physiology of chordal preservation. (**a**) The parallel bars are the mitral annulus. (**b**) The arms of the gymnasts are chordae and their bodies the papillary muscles. The floor is the left ventricular wall. (Reproduced with permission from *Indian J. Thorac. Cardiovasc. Surg.*)

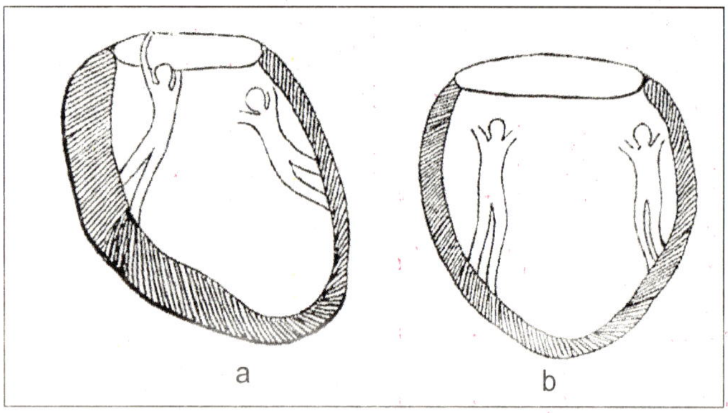

Fig. 1.43: Effect of chordal resection. Note dilatation and ventricular wall thickness where chordae are resected partially or completely. (**a**) Partial chordal resection, (**b**) complete chordal resection. (Reproduced with permission from *Indian. J. Thorac. Cardiovasc. Surg.*)

Technique (Miki's technique)

This technique is useful even in the most heavily calcified valves. With adequate exposure an incision is made in the belly of the anterior mitral leaflet at the 12 O'clock position a mm or two from the annulus and parallel to it (Figs 1.44, 1.45). This incision is extended towards the commissures on both sides. Two stay sutures are placed on the mitral annulus at 3 O'clock and 9 O'clock position and pulled up to the drapes. With blunt and sharp dissection the commissural fusion is divided and the anterior mitral leaflet is separated from the posterior mitral leaflet. The incision in the subvalvular apparatus is extended into the papillary muscle up to its base. The anterior mitral leaflet is now grasped with a right-angled clamp. Using a no. 11 knife, the chordae from the anterior papillary muscle is carefully shaved from the anterior mitral leaflet (Figs 1.46, 1.47). This is now resutured to the mitral annulus at the 10 O'clock position with a braided 2-0 suture. Similarly, the posterior papillary muscle chordae to anterior mitral leaflet are separated and resutured to the mitral annulus at the 12 O'clock position. The rest of the anterior mitral leaflet is excised (Figs 1.48, 1.49).

A curved hook is passed behind the posterior papillary muscle chordae to the posterior mitral leaflet. All fibrous and calcific material from the posterior mitral leaflet now comes into view and can be shaved leaving the chordae attached to the annulus with a thin remnant of the posterior mitral leaflet (Figs 1.50, 1.51). A similar shaving is performed on the chordae from the anterior papillary muscle to posterior mitral leaflet. The posterior mitral leaflet is now slit vertically from free edge to the annulus at the 6 O'clock position. Additional slits can be made at 4 O'clock and 7 O'clock positions if required. The left ventricle and left atrium are carefully washed several times with saline in a bulb syringe to remove any calcific or fibrous debris from there. The two sutures fixing the anterior mitral leaflet chordae are now tied. The mitral orifice will now accommodate any reasonably large valve. Any

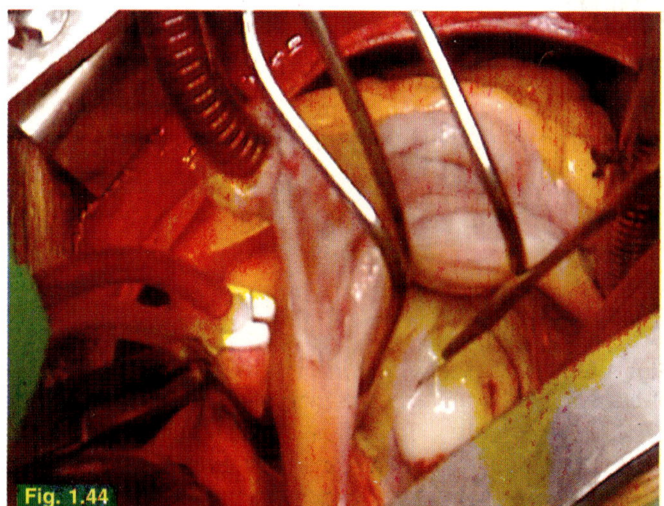

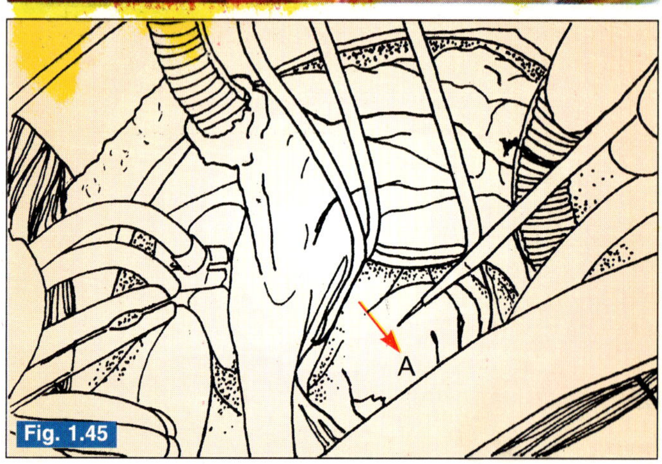

Figs 1.44, 1.45: Incision in the belly of the anterior mitral leaflet, the first step in excising the mitral valve.

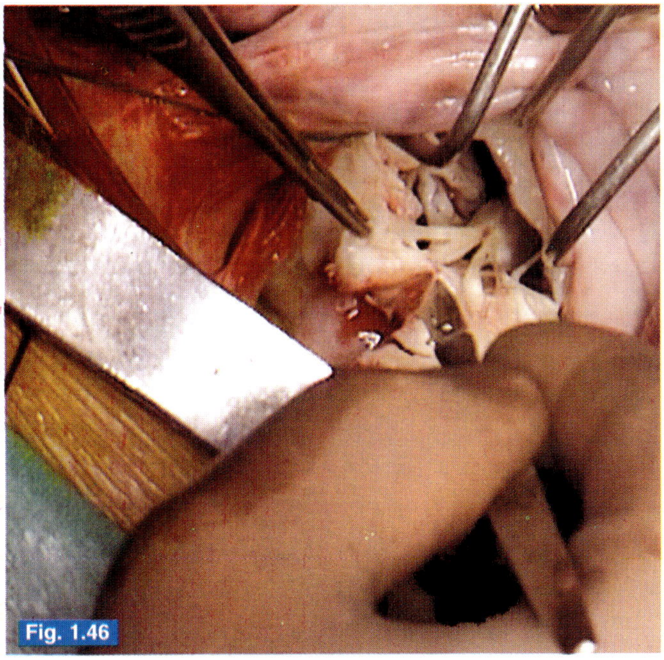

Fig. 1.46

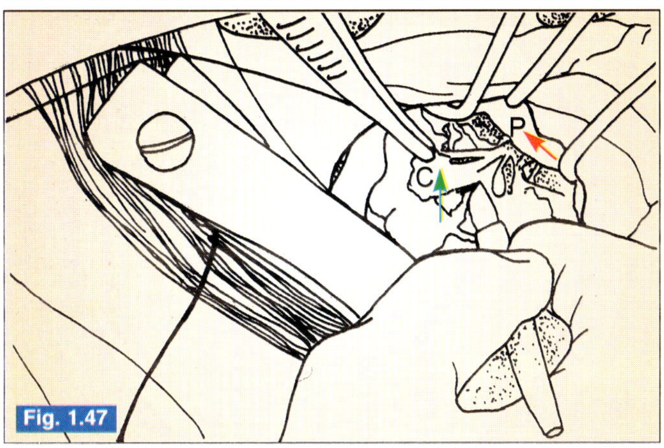

Fig. 1.47

Figs 1.46, 1.47: Technique of chordal preservation. Separation of the anterior mitral leaflet chordae (C) splitting down to the papillary muscle (P).

residual calcium can now be easily visualised and excised. Slit in the papillary muscles can be extended further if necessary. Careful attention must be paid to any loose tissue or chordal tag hanging free in the left ventricular cavity and must be excised.

There are several other techniques for full chordal preservation. These include the Feiki, David, Khonsari, etc. in which the anterior leaflet chordae are variously dealt with. We have found that the Miki technique described here is suitable for all (100%) of patients who require mitral valve replacement.

Sizing

Correct sizing of the annulus is very important (Fig. 1.52). A large size valve (31 mm St. Jude) has an orifice area of 5.18 cm^2. This will provide the patient an adequate effective orifice area for full exercise performance with low gradients. This may also provide free forward flow and reduce the possibility of thrombus formation. With experience nearly all patients can receive a reasonably large mitral valve prosthesis (29 or 31 mm St. Jude). The surgeon's attitude and desire to provide the patient a large effective orifice area is the most important factor in valve sizing.

Valve Suture

The author has used a horizontal interrupted mattress technique for more than 3 decades in nearly 4000 mitral valve replacements. This technique will be described.

Use of pledgeted sutures is best discouraged for routine use. They add additional foreign material and provide a nidus for thrombus formation. Pledgeted

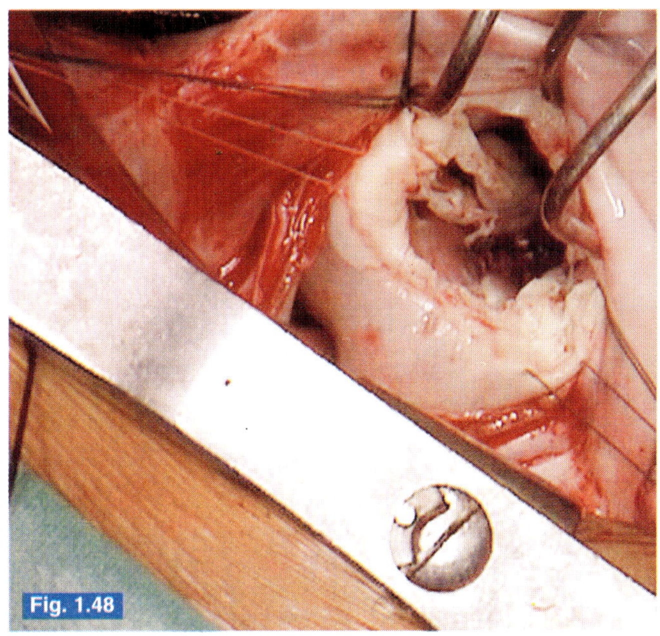

Fig. 1.48

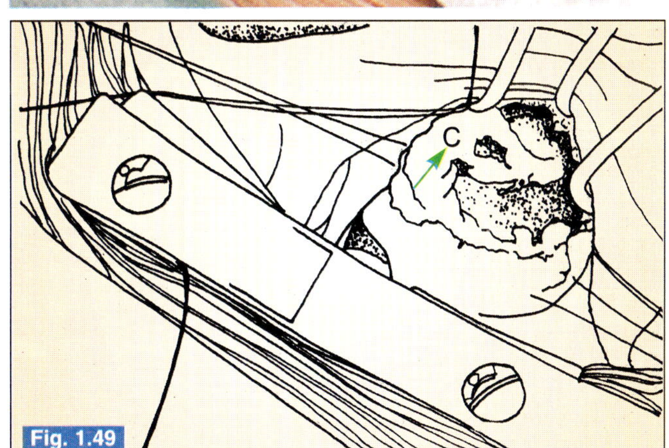

Fig. 1.49

Figs 1.48, 1.49: Fixing the separated anterior leaflet chordal (C) to the mitral annulus. Note the location of the suture.

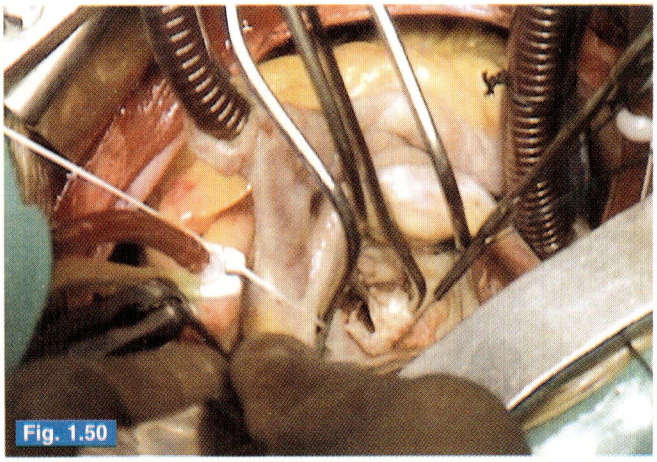

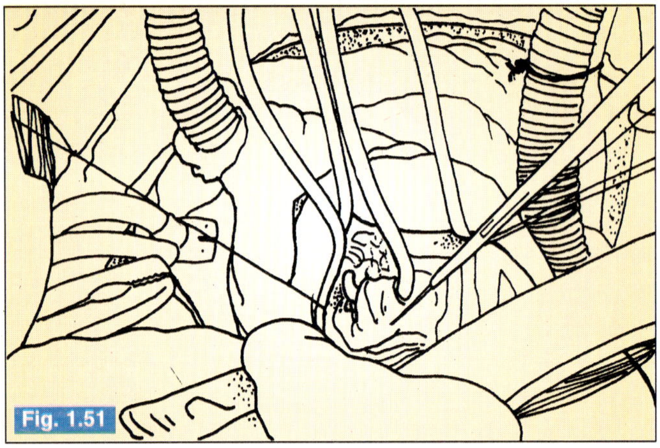

Figs 1.50, 1.51: Calcium from the posterior mitral leaflet is shaved, preserving the chordae.

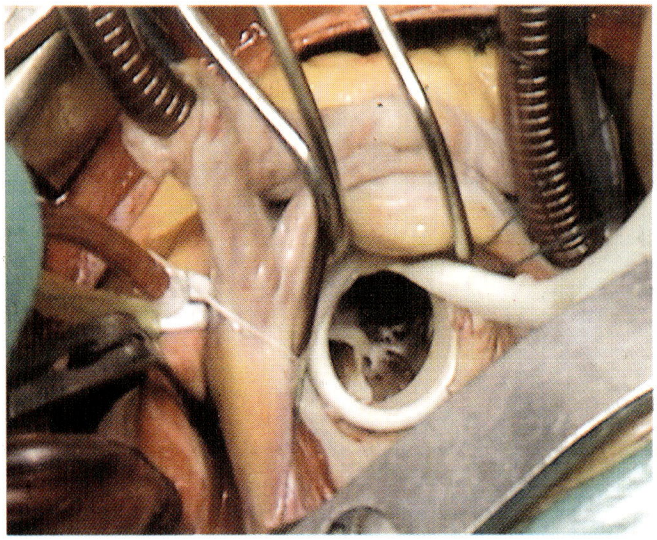

Fig. 1.52: Sizing of the mitral annulus after chordal preservation.

sutures may be required only rarely. A continuous 3-0 polypropylene suture (2–3) is used by some surgeons. Again, there is a higher risk of dehiscence and paravalvular leaks with this technique.

After sizing the mitral orifice an appropriate mechanical valve is obtained and mounted on a holder. Nonrotatable valves must be oriented properly before commencing the suture. The assistant holds the valve holder on the surgeon's side of the retractor. Proper orientation of the valve orifice must be checked at this time.

The first suture (25 mm needle, 2-0 ethibond) is passed at the 12 O'clock position from the atrial to the ventricular side of the sewing rim of the prosthesis (Figs 1.53, 1.54). These needles are now passed from the left ventricle to left atrial side of the patient's mitral valve annulus. This provides an everting suture line. The next 2 sutures are placed in similar fashion at 11 and 10 O'clock positions. These sutures can also gather up the remnant of the chordae fixed earlier to the annulus. Suture no. 4 and 5 are placed at the 1 and 2 O'clock positions. The distance between the threads of each suture and between the sutures must be uniform and should

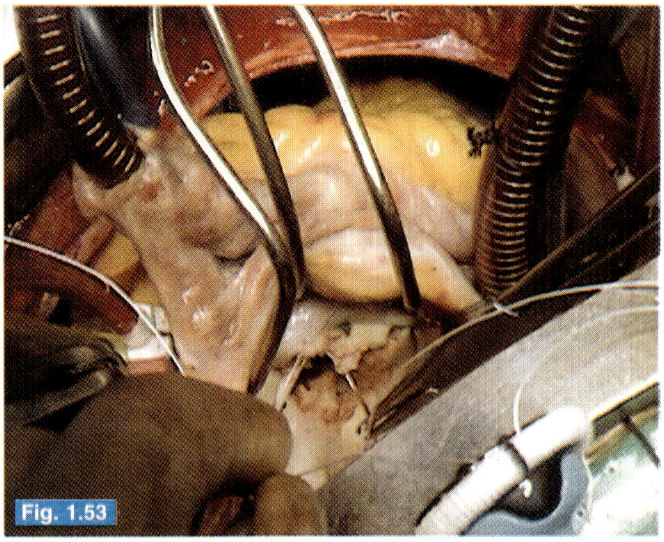

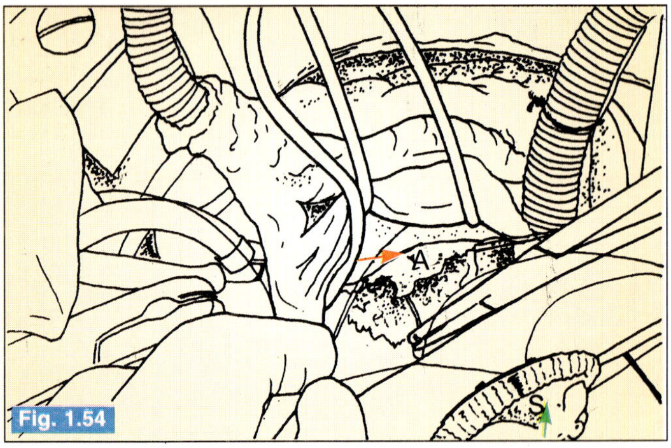

Figs 1.53, 1.54: Technique of implantation of the mitral valve. The first double-armed suture is passed backhand through the sewing ring (S) and then through the anterior mitral annulus (A) everting it.

cover the anterior half of mitral annulus from 9 O'clock to 3 O'clock position.

The assistant now shifts the valve holder to his right hand and moves the prosthesis to the left side of the sternal retractor. Again, alternate white and green sutures are taken in everting fashion beginning at the 6 O'clock position on the prosthesis (Figs 1.55, 1.56). The posterior mitral leaflet is plicated placing tension on the chordae of the posterior mitral leaflet with 5 sutures. These cover the posterior half of mitral annulus between the 9 and 3 O'clock positions. The sutures are held taut and the valve holder is pushed down to position the prosthesis in the annulus. The holder is removed and all sutures are tied. The 12 and 6 O'clock sutures are retained on haemostats. The remaining sutures are tied and cut. The valve disc (discs) orientation and free movement are checked several times. The valve is now rotated (if rotatable) for at least one full circle to ensure that no suture or tissue entanglement exists (Figs 1.57, 1.58). It is checked again from free movement of the disc (discs) in the correct direction. A Foley catheter

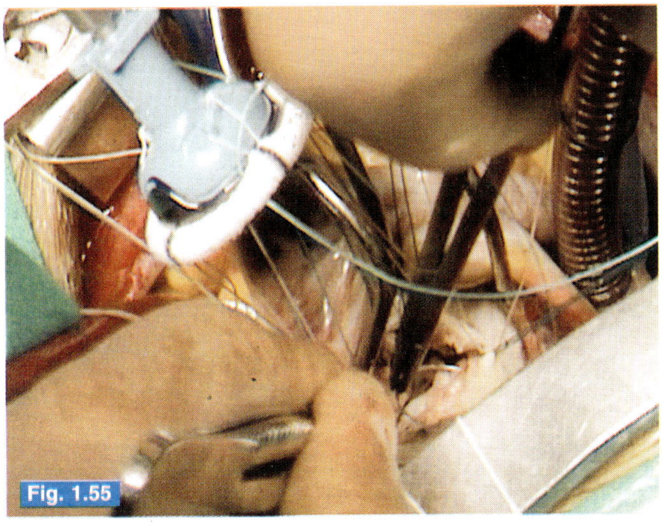

Fig. 1.55

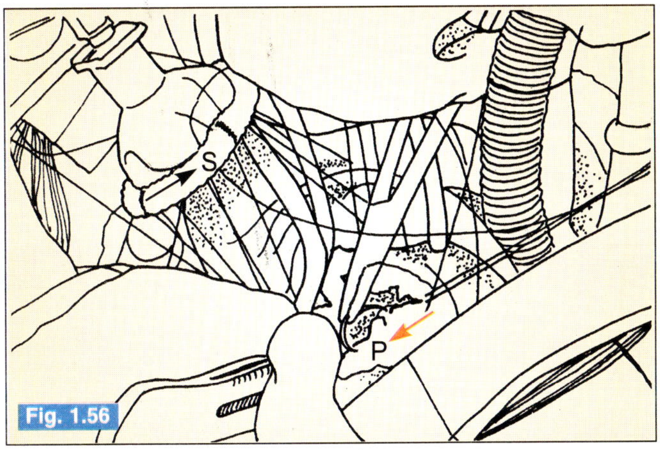

Fig. 1.56

Figs 1.55, 1.56: Technique of suturing the mitral valve. The double-armed suture passes first through the sewing ring (S) and then through the posterior mitral annulus (P) everting it.

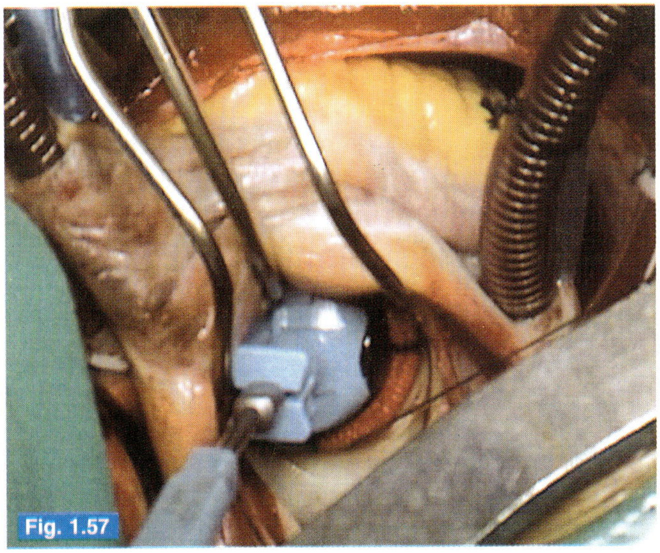

Fig. 1.57

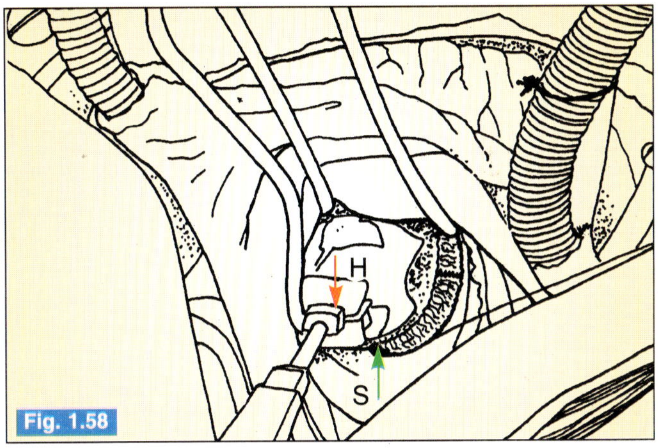

Fig. 1.58

Figs 1.57, 1.58: Rotation of the mechanical mitral valve within the sewing ring (S) with the holder (H).

is passed through the valve (between the discs) and the bulb is inflated to keep the prosthesis incompetent (Fig. 1.59).

Mitral Valve Replacement Through Aorta

The mitral annulus is sized (Fig. 1.60). In this approach the mounted mitral mechanical valve is first oriented properly and held by an assistant. The posterior annular sutures are placed first. As before these are double-armed braided sutures with 25 mm half circle (or 17 mm) sutures. In order to locate the knots on the atrial side (everting sutureline) the lower half or posterior annular sutures are placed first (Figs 1.61, 1.62). The needles pass from the atrial side of the sewing rim into the ventricular side. These then pass from the left ventricular to left atrial side plicating the posterior mitral leaflet. When 5 sutures are placed, the valve is lowered into the mitral annulus (without the holder) and the sutures are tied on the atrial side. The anterior half of the prosthesis is now pushed into the left atrium and sutured to the anterior mitral

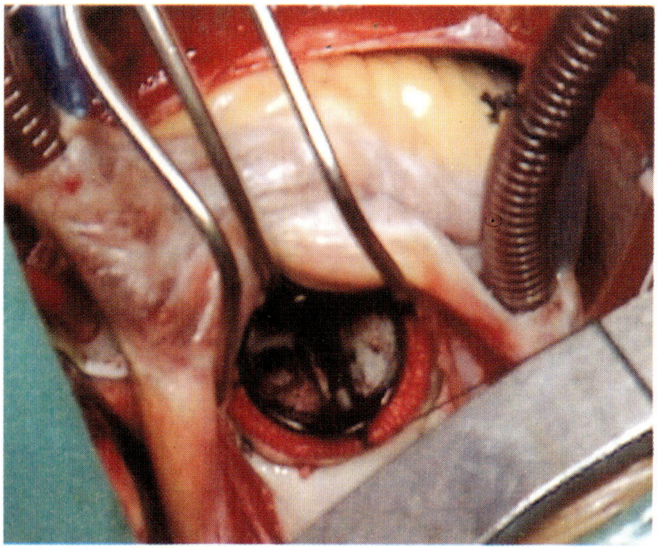

Fig. 1.59: Completed mitral valve replacement with a mechanical valve. Note the orientation of the discs.

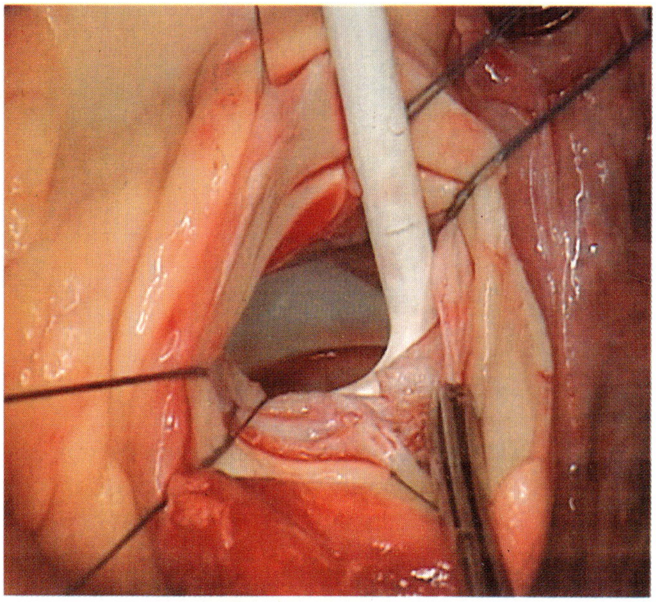

Fig. 1.60: Sizing the mitral valve annulus through the aorta.

annulus (Figs 1.63, 1.64). When these are tied and cut, the valve orientation is once again checked carefully (Figs 1.64, 1.65). The retained 6 O'clock and 12 O'clock sutures are used to steady the valve while it is rotated carefully.

Tissue Valve Implantation

Once the size of tissue valve for implantation is decided, the appropriate valve is obtained and rinsed by agitating for 3 minutes each (total 6 min) in two bowls of sterile saline or ringer lactate. This is to remove the gluteraldehyde from the valve. .It takes full six minutes for this procedure.

Preparation for Implantation

The tissue valve struts may: (a) Obstruct the left ventricular outflow tract, (b) may entangle the suture, and (c) the valve is not rotatable. A few details must be carefully observed for proper and successful

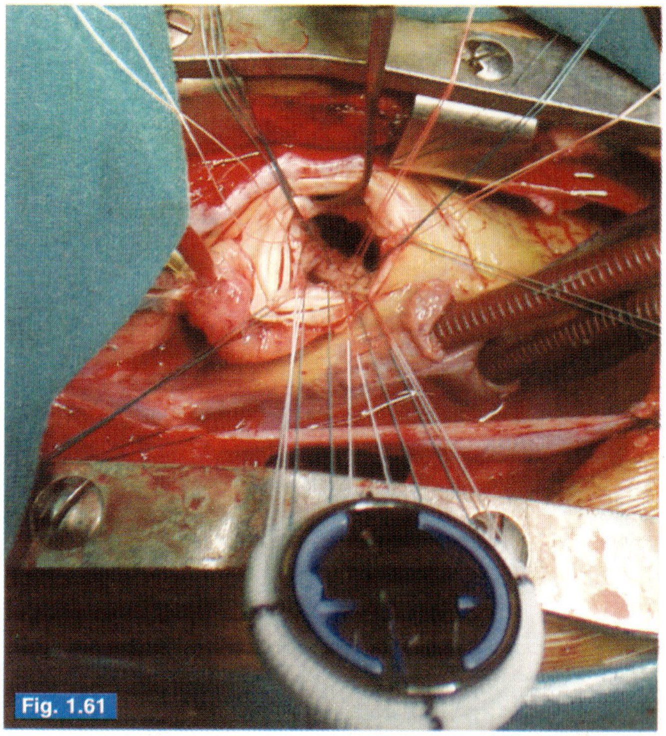

Fig. 1.61

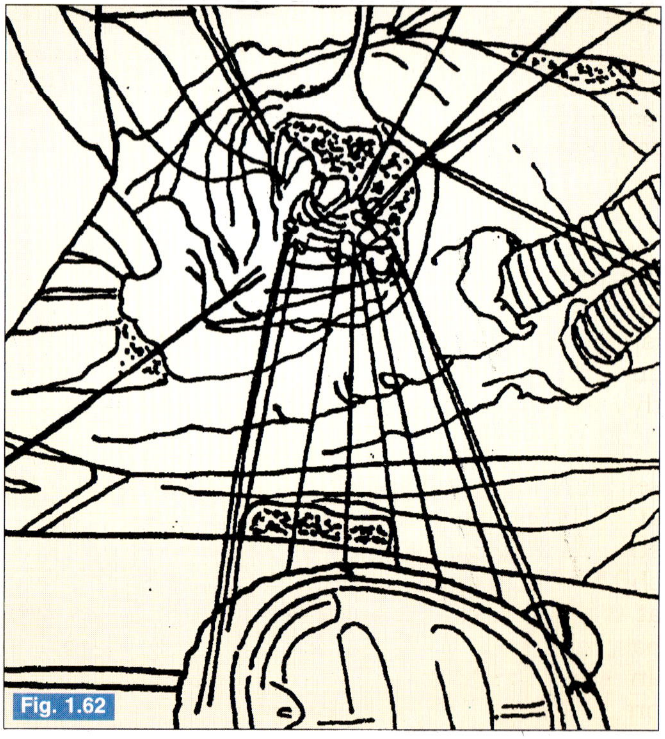

Fig. 1.62

Figs 1.61, 1.62: Technique of mitral valve implantation through the aorta. Placement of sutures for the posterior mitral annulus.

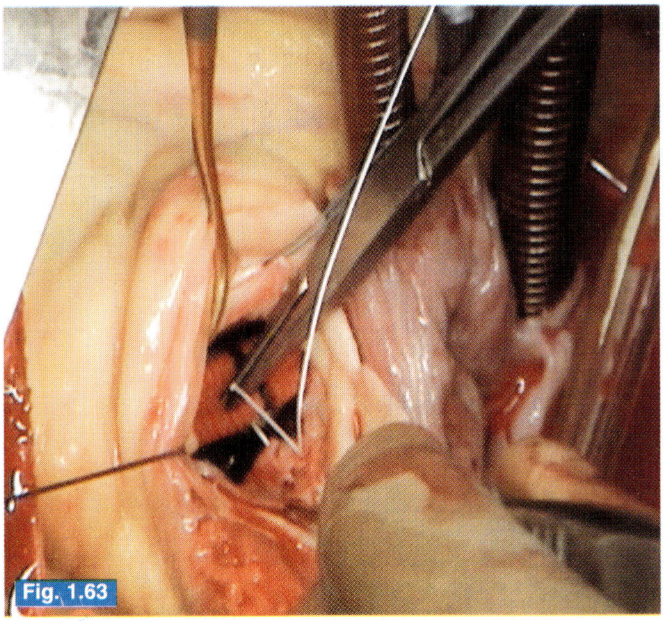

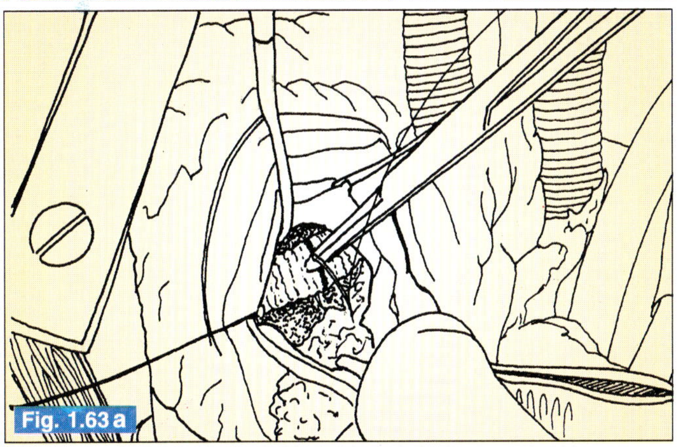

Figs 1.63, 1.63 a: The last suture for the mitral valve replacement through the aorta, from the sewing rim to the anterior annulus.

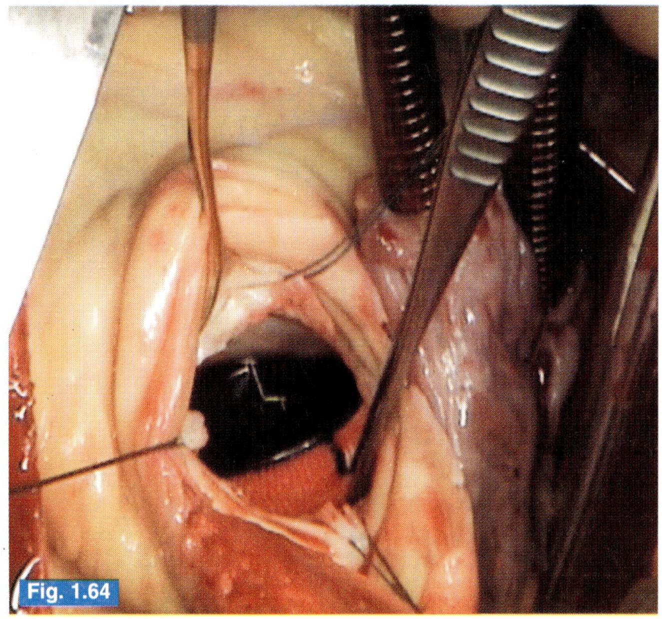

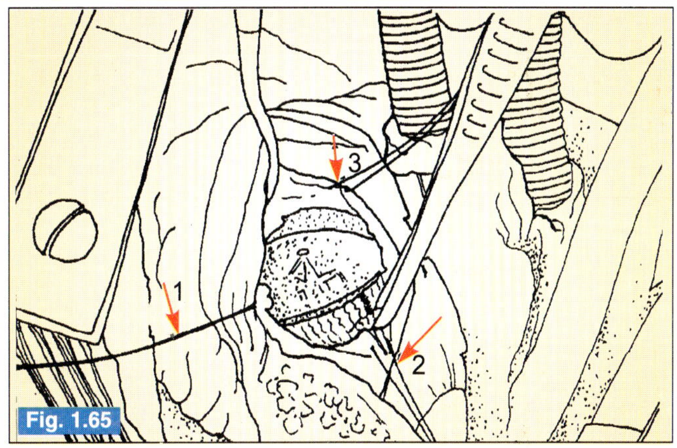

Figs 1.64, 1.65: Completed implantation of the mitral valve through the aorta; 1, 2 and 3 are the aortic commissural stay sutures.

implantation of the valve. When the handle is inserted into the holder it is tightened gently until it is fully tightened. This will tense the green sutures anchoring the holder to the valve and also retract the 3 struts inwards preventing suture entanglement.

There are two black line markers on the cloth sewing rim (Figs 1.66, 1.67). These should be oriented at 9 O'clock and 12 O'clock positions to avoid the strut form causing left ventricular outflow tract obstruction. To do this the first suture is taken the at the 12 O'clock position on the sewing rim and passed through the 12 O'clock position on the mitral annulus. The valve is now ready for implantation in proper orientation.

The valve is then held by the assistant just as he does for the mechanical valve. The method for suturing is identical to that used for mechanical valve. However, while lowering the valve into the mitral orifice the sutures are retracted sideways with a silk tie. The silk tie is passed around 3 or 4 sutures at the struts and held on haemostats (Figs 1.68, 1.69). This will prevent suture entanglements in the struts when the valve is lowered into the left ventricular cavity. Once all 3 struts are fully into the left ventricle the sutures are pulled tight. The silk tie is removed and the sutures are tied and divided. The holder remains in situ till now. Three green sutures anchoring the holder are now divided and the holder is withdrawn and inspected for complete removal of the anchoring sutures. The left ventricular cavity is filled with saline to observe for proper coaptation of the three cusps and for any paravalvular leaks (Figs 1.70–1.71).

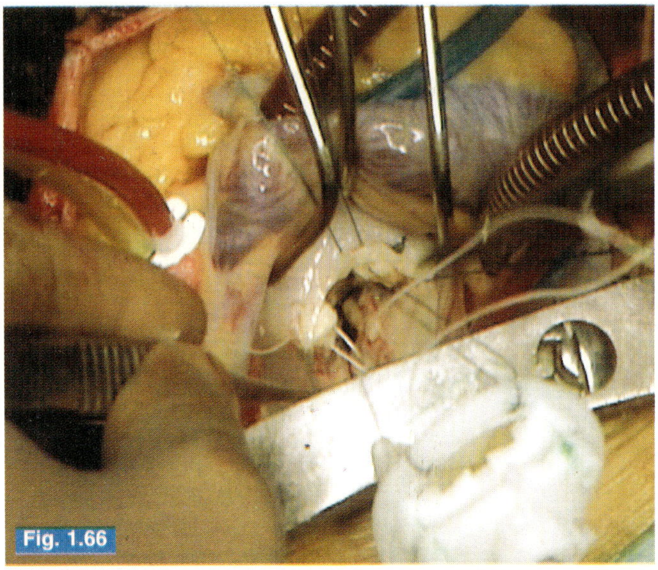

Fig. 1.66

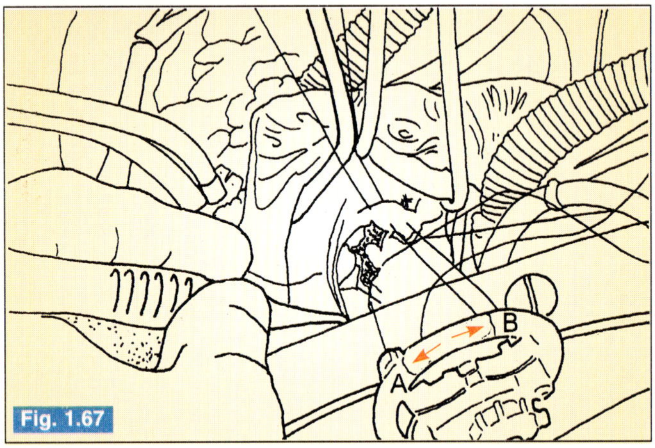

Fig. 1.67

Figs 1.66, 1.67: Tissue valve orientation and suturing. Note the two black marks on the sewing rim (A and B) and their relative position on the mitral annulus to prevent the strut obstructing the aortic outflow.

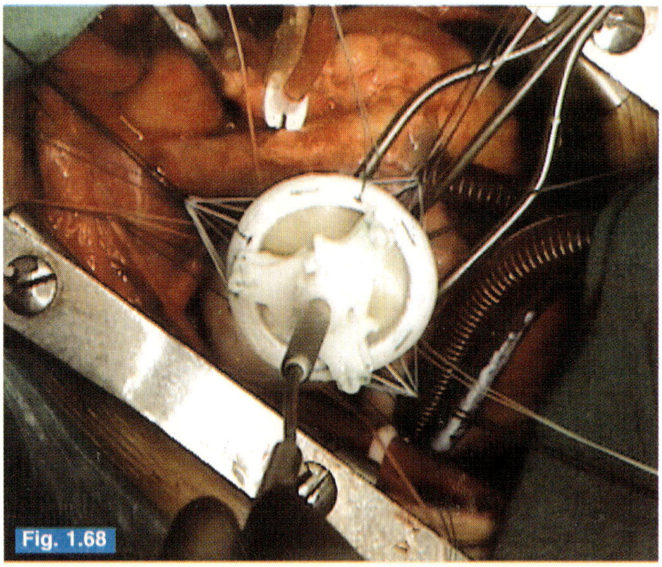

Fig. 1.68

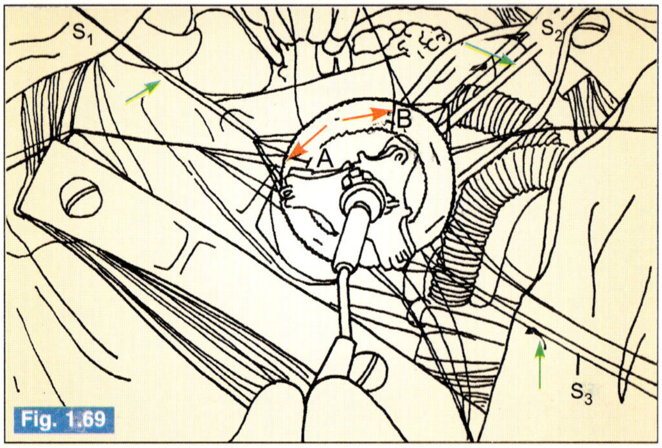

Fig. 1.69

Figs 1.68, 1.69: Traction on the sutures by the silk loop (S_1, S_2 and S_3) to prevent them from entangling in the struts. Note the two black lines on the sewing rim at 10 O'clock and 12 O'clock positions (A and B).

Implantation of the Autograft

Preparation

A decision to use the pulmonary autograft is made after transesophageal echocardiography. The pulmonary valve morphology and function are seen on the 2-D echo and the annulus is measured.

Because of pulmonary hypertension the pulmonary annulus generally measures between 26–30 mm and is ideally suited for this purpose. In addition, pulmonary arterial hypertension causes right ventricular hypertrophy making harvesting the pulmonary autograft easier and less hazardous to the first septal artery (Fig. 1.72). Also the pulmonary arterial wall is thicker and the valve cusps are conditioned to withstand higher pressures.

Before cardiopulmonary bypass is established the pulmonary artery is separated from the aorta by blunt and sharp dissection (Figs 1.73, 1.74). It is then looped carefully avoiding any injury to the left main coronary artery and aorta. A marker suture (4.0 braided / 5-0 polypropylene) is placed on the pulmonary artery just distal to the sinus. This will ensure that no injury occurs to the pulmonary valve cusps or commissures when an incision is made.

Autograft Harvesting

When the mitral valve has been excised and chordal preservation is completed, the Cooley atrial retractor is removed.

An incision is made in the pulmonary artery just distal to the marker suture. The pulmonary artery is now divided transversely halfway through the circumference (Figs 1.75, 1.76). The pulmonary valve is inspected for its morphology and structure. It

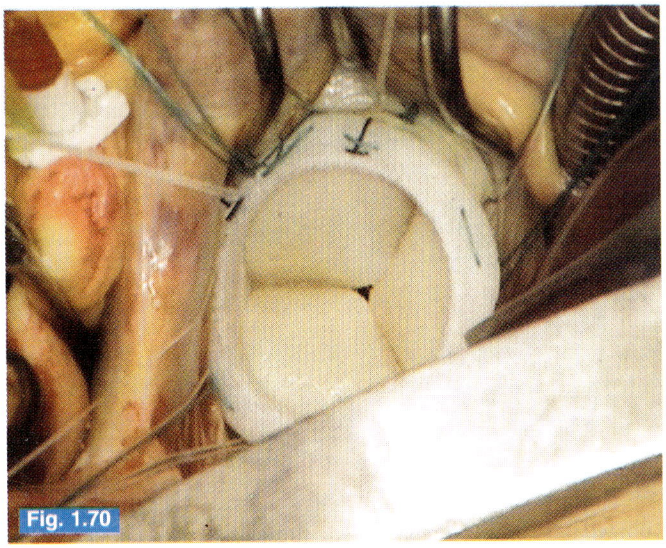

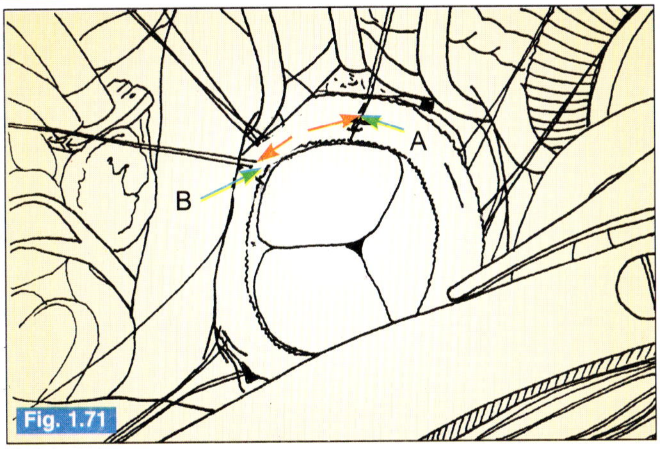

Figs 1.70, 1.71: The completed tissue valve implantation. Note the two markers at 12 O'clock (A) and 10 O'clock (B) position.

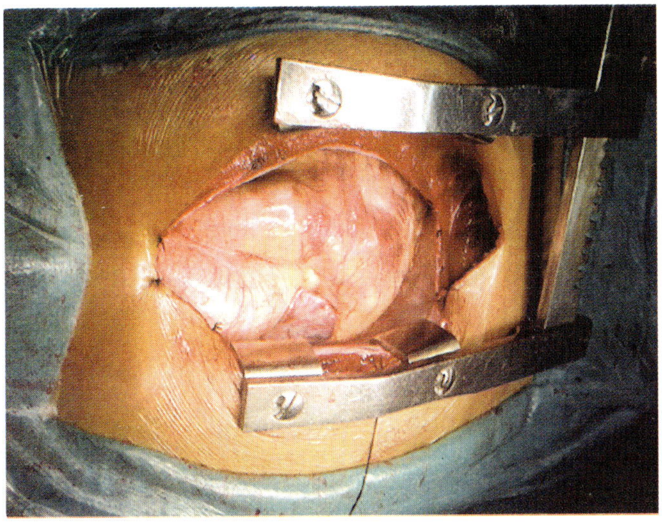

Fig. 1.72: The heart. Note the enlarged pulmonary artery due to hypertension.

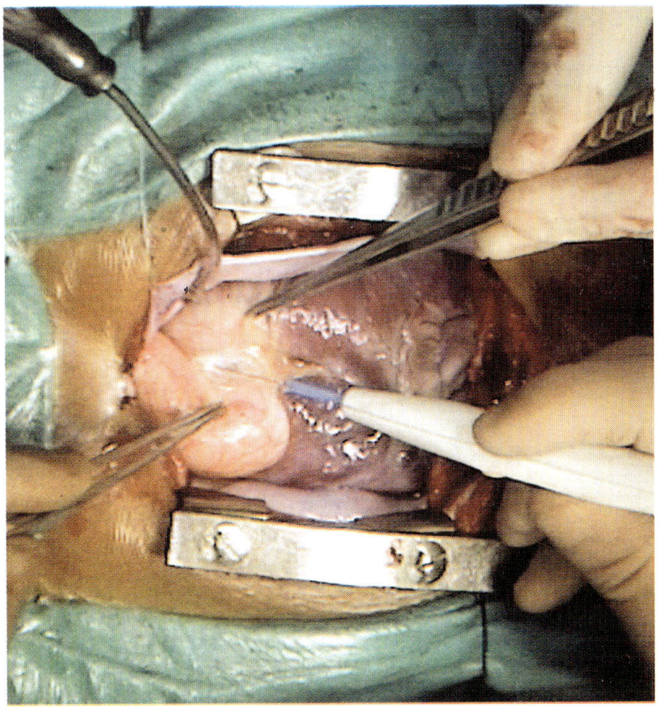

Fig. 1.73: Dissection of the pulmonary aorta junction to separate the two great arteries.

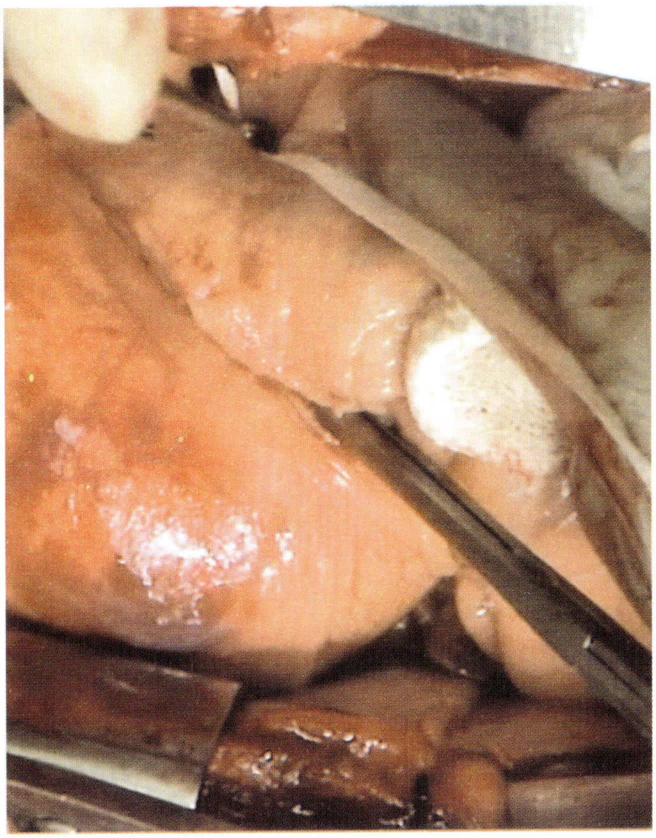

Fig. 1.74: Looping of the pulmonary artery.

should be tricuspid, with normal cusps without thickening, fusion or perforation. If any of these are seen, the procedure is abandoned and the pulmonary arterial incision is closed by suture. If it is normal then the pulmonary trunk is divided completely just 1 or 2 mm above the top of the valve commissures.

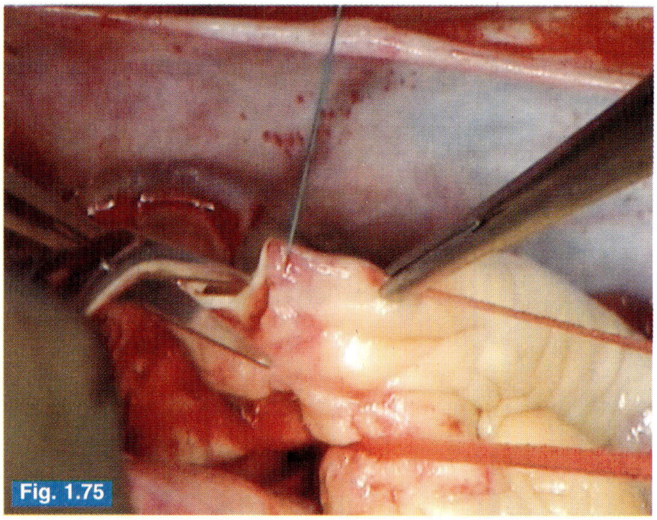

Fig. 1.75

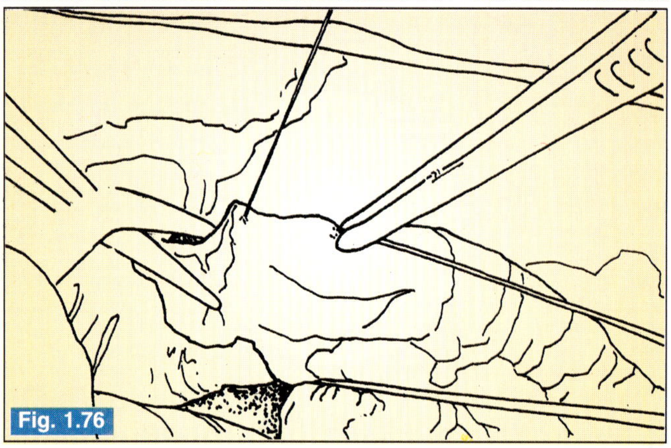

Fig. 1.76

Figs 1.75, 1.76: The first step in harvesting the autograft. Division of the pulmonary artery just beyond the marker stitch.

For safety a right-angled clamp is placed (by lifting the tape) behind the pulmonary artery (Figs 1.77, 1.78). When fully divided, it is carefully separated from the epicardial adhesions to the back of the right ventricular outflow tract.

A right-angled clamp is now introduced through the pulmonary valve into the right ventricular outflow tract and pushes the anterior right ventricular wall just below the valve. This is grasped on the epicardial side by forceps and a stab incision is made and deepened to enter the right ventricular cavity under vision to avoid any injury to the cusps (Fig. 1.79). The right ventricular outflow tract incision is extended circumferentially. Care must be taken to avoid injury to the left anterior descending branch to the left of this incision which should be curved backwards at this point. By careful dissection on the medial side the right ventricular outflow tract muscle is bevelled and shaved one or two mm's below the valve cusps. Here careful dissection will avoid injury to the right coronary sinus of the aorta and the right coronary artery. The assistant now retracts the autograft leftwards with a forceps. The dissection over the infundibular septum is bevelled to avoid producing a ventricular septal defect (Figs 1.80, 1.81). This dissection is carried leftwards until the first septal artery comes into view. This artery is carefully separated from the autograft. In patients with pulmonary hypertension this artery

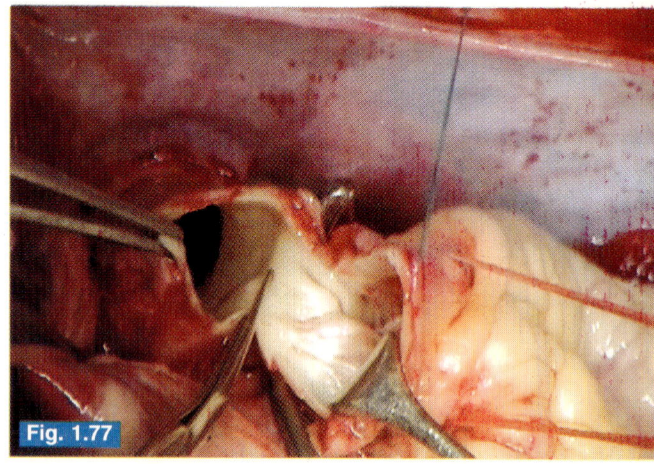

Fig. 1.77

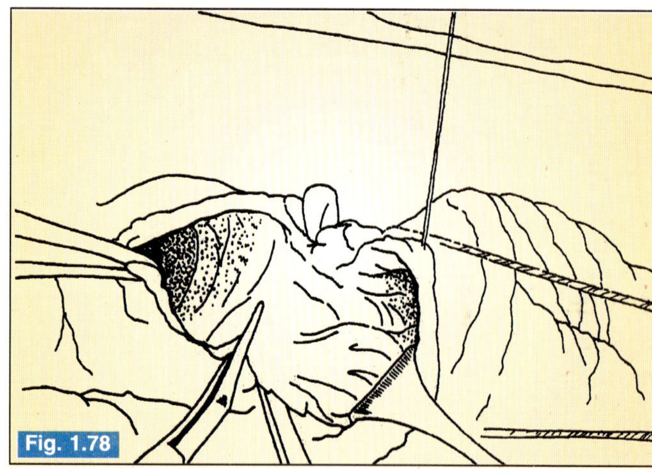

Fig. 1.78

Figs 1.77, 1.78: Division of the pulmonary artery. Note the clamp behind to prevent injury to the coronary arteries.

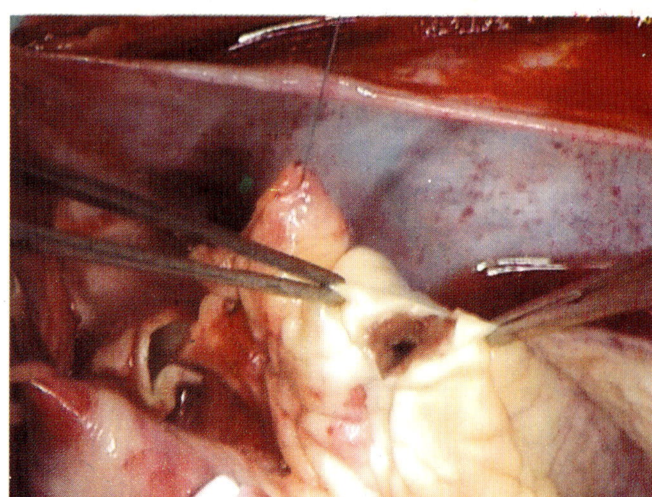

Fig. 1.79: The incision in the right ventricular outflow tract.

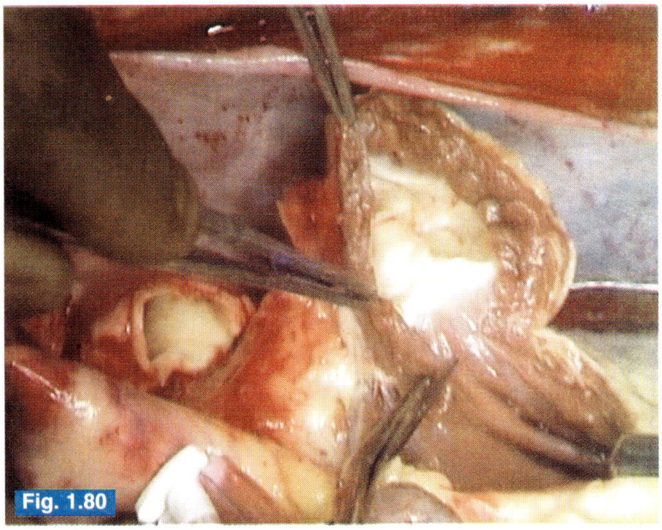
Fig. 1.80

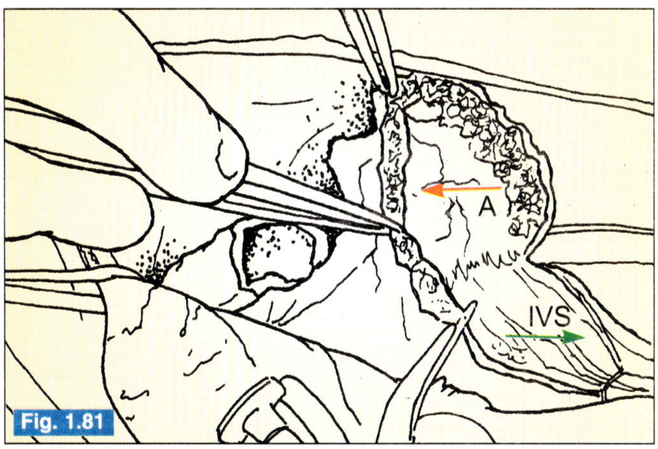

Fig. 1.81

Figs 1.80, 1.81: Dissection of the autograft (A) from the interventricular septum (IVS). Note the plane of dissection.

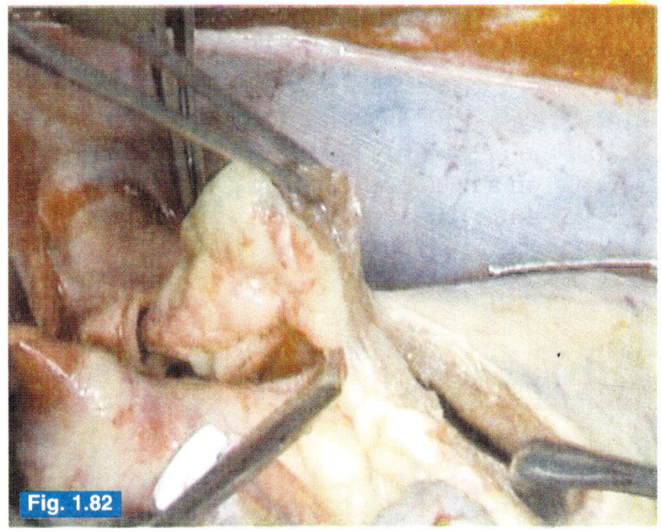
Fig. 1.82

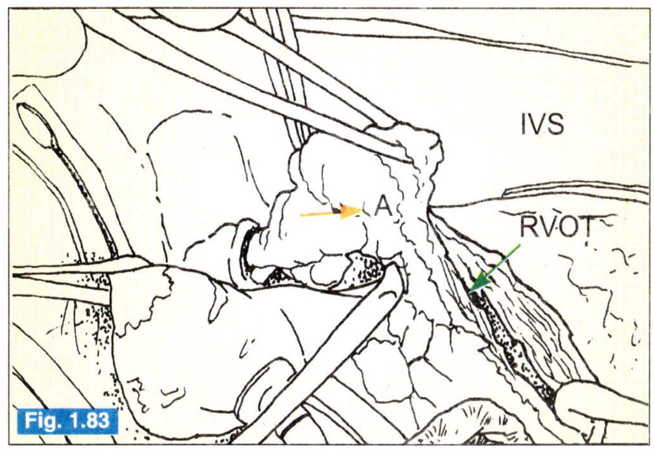

Fig. 1.83

Figs 1.82, 1.83: Separation of pulmonary autograft (A) from the right ventricular outflow tract (RVOT).

may not be seen because of the muscle hypertrophy. However, dissection can be learned in cadaver hearts before attempting on a patient. The dissection can also proceed from the left leaving a clear 2–3 mm rim of right ventricular outflow tract muscle away from the left anterior descending for anastomosis of the homograft later (Figs 1.82, 1.83). When the autograft is fully separated, it is held with forceps on the adventitial side of the pulmonary artery and inspected for any injury to the cusps (Fig. 1.84). It is then sized using a conical graduated sizer passed from below towards the pulmonary artery.

Autograft Implantation

This procedure requires precise orientation, proper suturing and a little artistic imagination for success.

Three 4-0 polypropylene sutures are passed through the tops of the commissural pillars at the distal pulmonary artery end of the autograft (Figs 1.85, 1.86). The double armed suture needles are passed from epicardial to endocardial side. The needles are then passed through the mitral annulus at 2 O'clock, 6 O'clock and 10 O'clock positions to orient the pulmonary valve commissures in a tricuspid fashion.

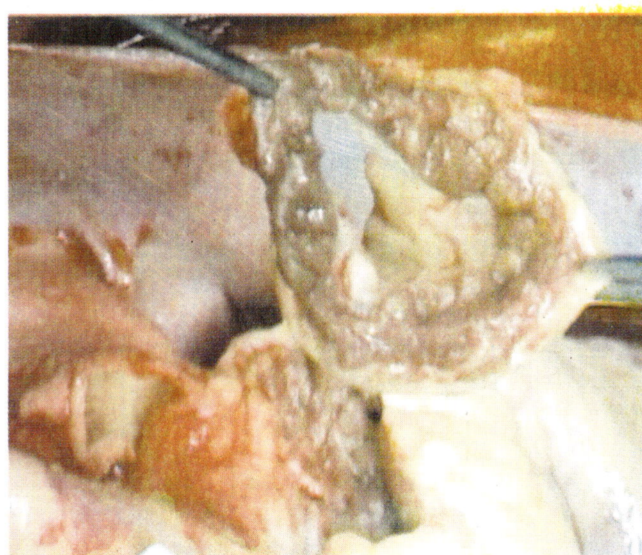

Fig. 1.84: The separated autograft is inspected.

The needles pass from the left ventricle to left atrial side of the annulus and are held on haemostats. Each suture is tied with at least 6 knots but is not divided. The autograft is now inverted into the left ventricular cavity. One needle from the 2 O'clock suture is now mounted on a needle holder and using a continuous suture technique the edge of the pulmonary artery is sutured to the mitral annulus in an anticlockwise direction (Figs 1.87, 1.88). On reaching the 10 O'clock suture it is tied to one strand and retained on a haemostat for later identification of the commissural location. Using the second needle the suture now proceeds from 10 O'clock to 6 O'clock and back to the 2 O'clock position in an identical manner. In this way the pulmonary artery end of the autograft is sutured to the mitral annulus (Figs 1.89, 1.90). The remnants of these sutures identify the location of the commissural pillars of the autograft valve.

A piece of Teflon felt previously fashioned for this purpose as shown in the figure is taken and held on a haemostat. The circumference of the base of this tripod felt stent is the circumference of the pulmonary autograft. The height of the struts is the height of the pulmonary artery sinus measured before cardiopulmonary bypass (Figs 1.91, 1.92).

The three commissural sutures are now passed through the top of these strut pillars of the Teflon felt stent. The free end of the base is now closed by a 5-0 polypropylene suture (Figs 1.93, 1.94). The commissural sutures are tied and cut fixing the felt stent to the mitral annulus. The autograft is now everted carefully into the left atrium through the stent (Figs 1.95, 1.96).

The 4-0 polypropylene double armed sutures are used for the proximal sutureline within the left atrium. The first suture passes at the base of the commissural triangle of the pulmonary autograft (at the 2 O'clock position), the needles pass through the base of the teflon felt stent and are passed through the endocardium of the left atrium about 2 cm upstream

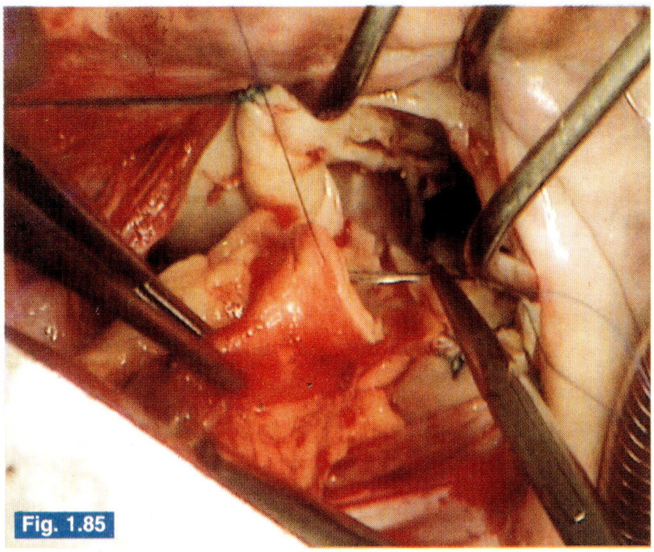

Fig. 1.85

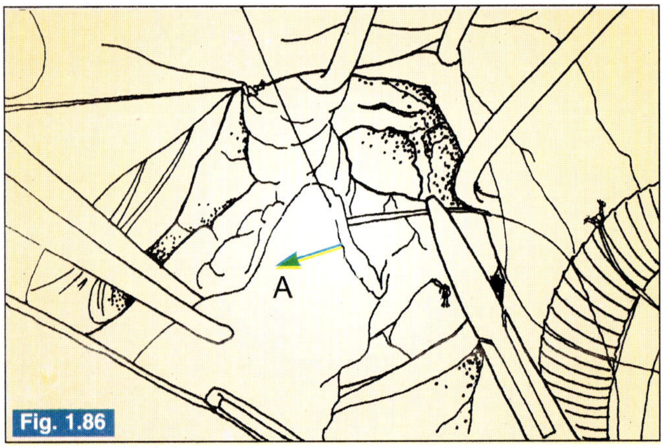

Fig. 1.86

Figs 1.85, 1.86: Location of commissural sutures on the pulmonary autograft (A).

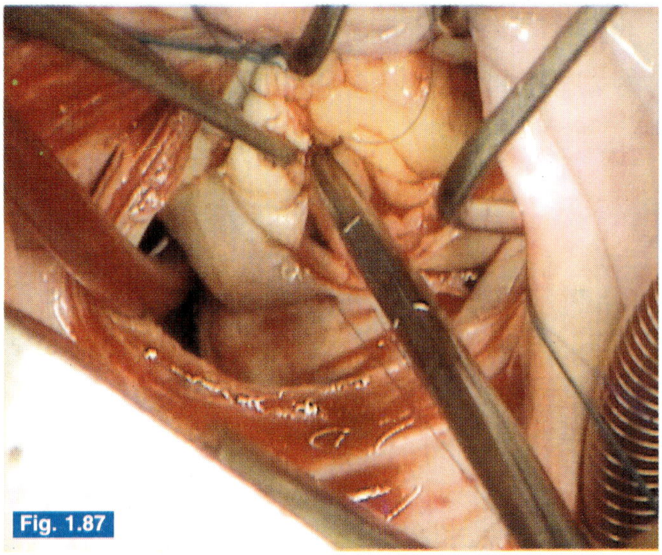

Fig. 1.87

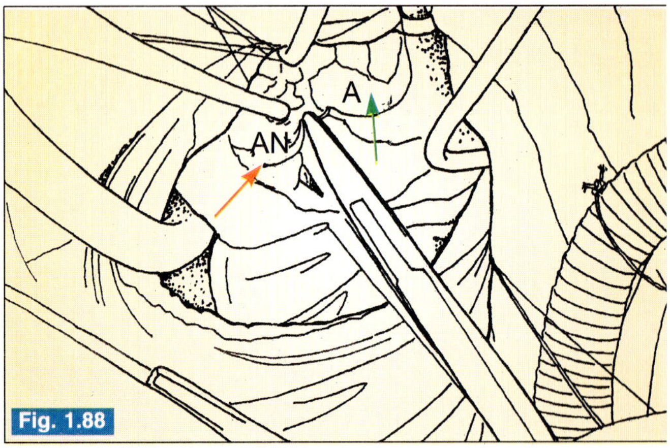

Fig. 1.88

Figs 1.87, 1.88: Pulmonary autograft (A) suture to the mitral annulus (AN) posterior aspect. Note the autograft is inverted into the left ventricle.

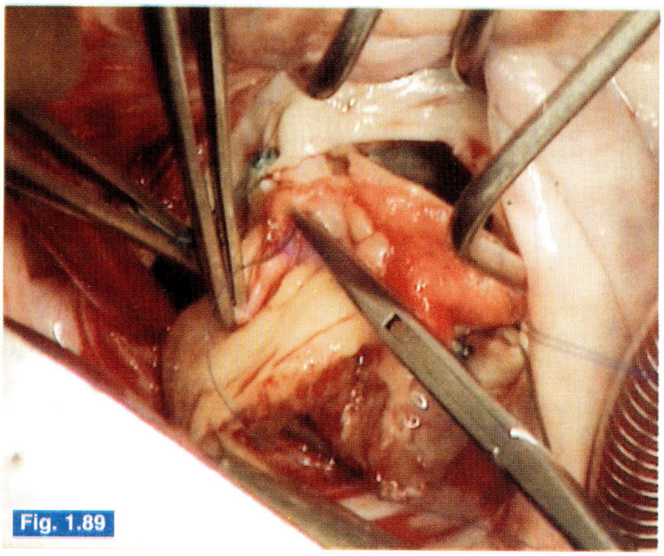
Fig. 1.89

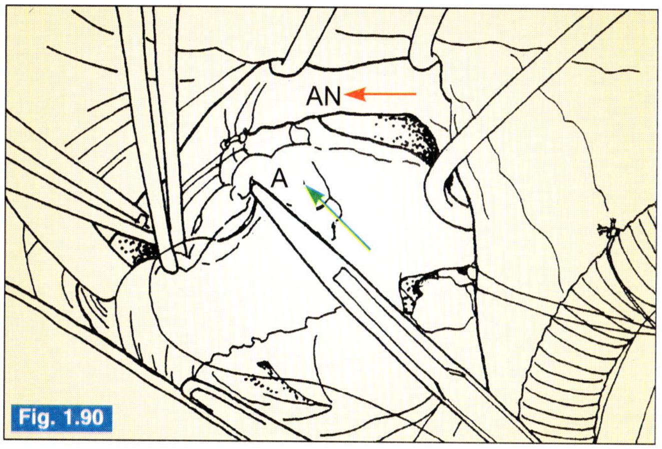

Fig. 1.90

Figs 1.89, 1.90: Pulmonary autograft (A) suture to the mitral annulus (AN) anterior aspect.

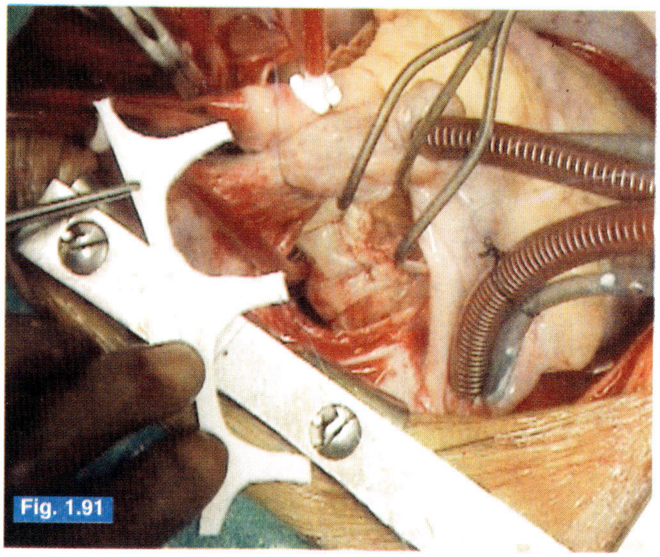
Fig. 1.91

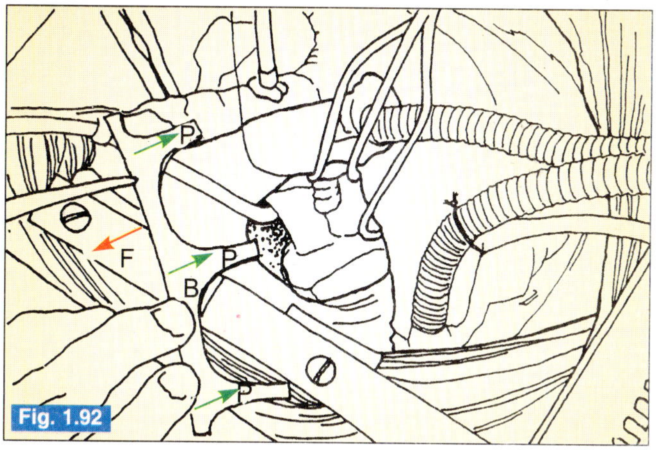

Fig. 1.92

Figs 1.91, 1.92: The tripod teflon felt (F) scaffold. Each pillar (P) is sutured to the commissural point (see text), the base (B) forms the ring.

of the mitral annulus (Figs 1.97, 1.98). Similarly two other sutures anchor the muscular proximal end of the autograft just below the commissural triangles at the 6 O'clock and 10 O'clock positions as well. These needles pass through the felt stent and gather up the endocardium of the left atrium again about 2 cm

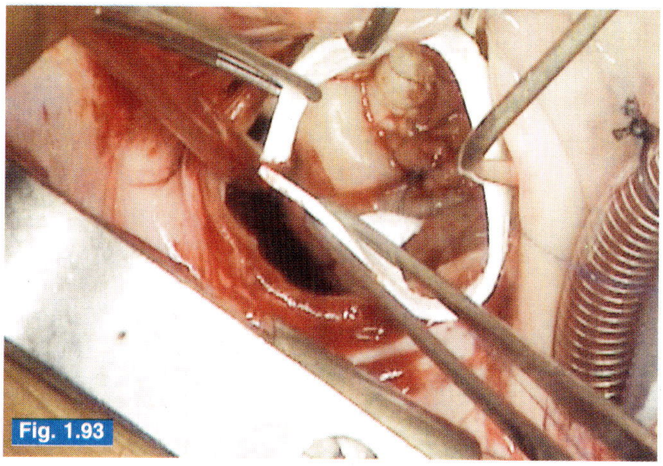
Fig. 1.93

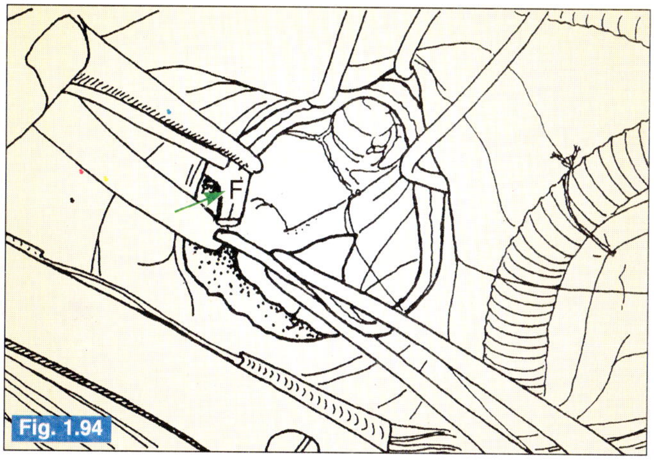

Fig. 1.94

Figs 1.93, 1.94: Closing the teflon felt scaffold (F) as a completed ring.

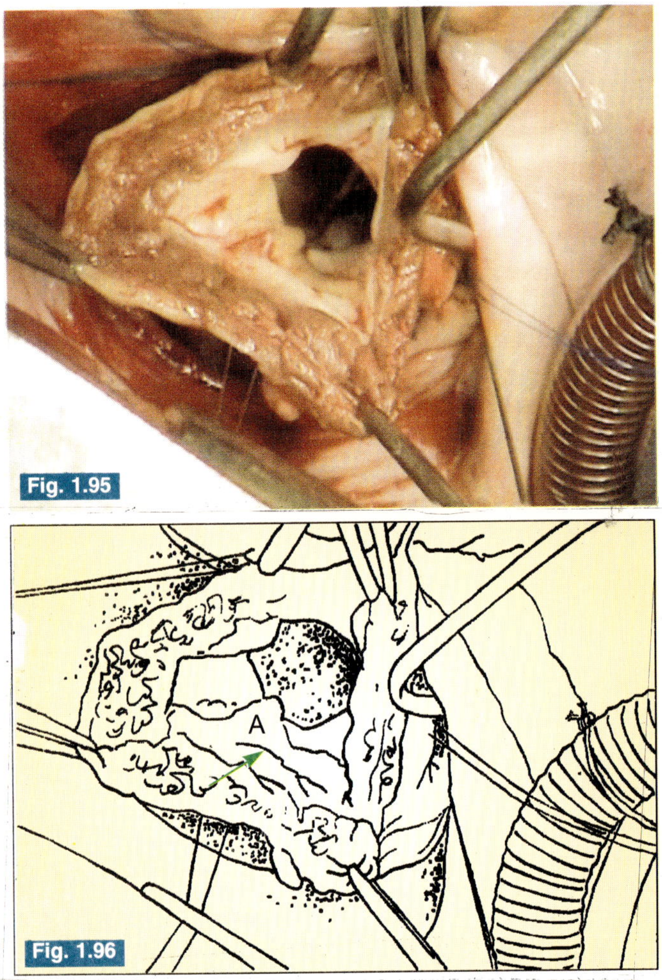

Figs 1.95, 1.96: The pulmonary autograft (A) everted into the left atrium after the distal end is sutured to the mitral annulus.

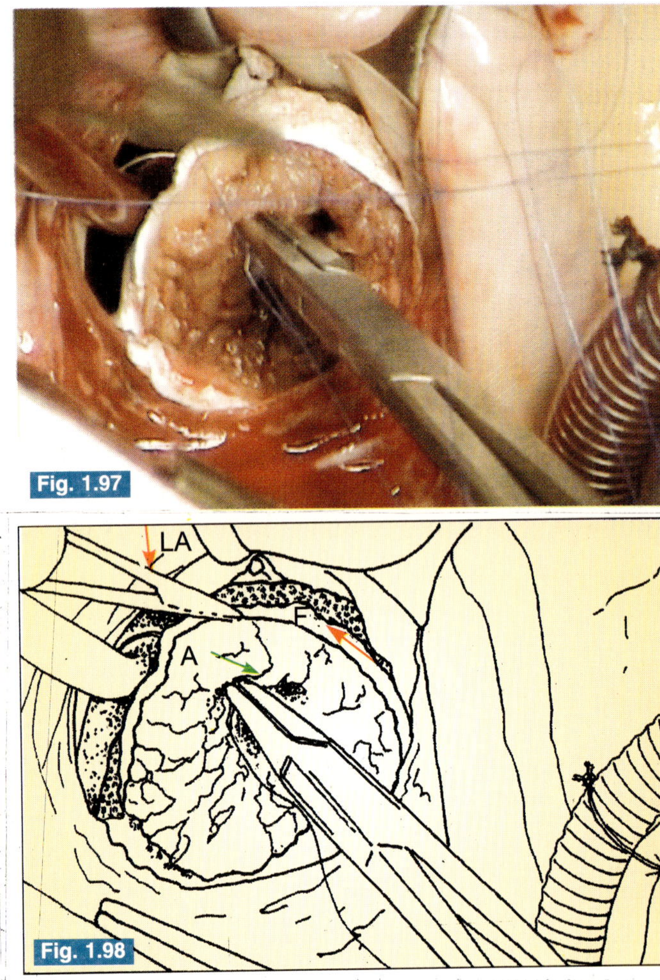

Figs 1.97, 1.98: Technique of pulmonary autograft (A), suture in the left atrium (LA), teflon felt (F) scaffold. The needle passes from inside the autograft outwards.

upstream of the mitral annulus (Figs 1.99, 1.100). In this way the tube of the pulmonary autograft is anchored in the left atrium, with the teflon felt stent which is buried between the autograft and left atrial wall, supporting it from collapsing (Figs 1.101, 1.102). Three other sutures of 4-0 polypropylene anchor the autograft to the left atrial wall midway between the commissures. All sutures are tied. They are then run

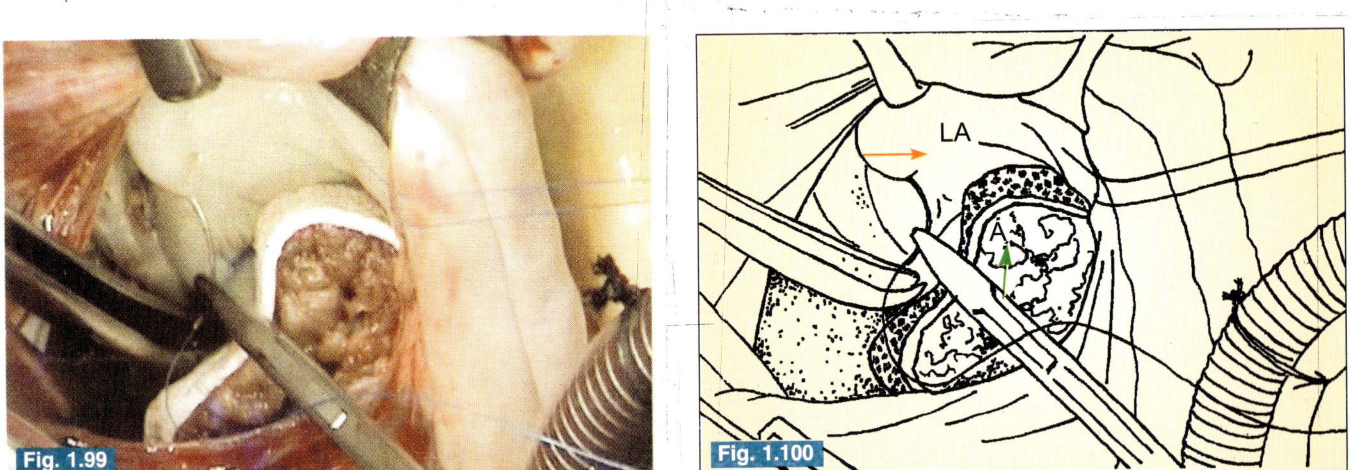

Figs 1.99, 1.100: Suturing the pulmonary autograft (A) in the left atrium (LA).

in a continuous fashion obliterating any space between the autograft and left atrial wall. In this way the autograft is supported by the teflon felt stent and is located wholly in the left atrial cavity. The valve is now tested by injecting saline through the autograft into the left ventricle (Figs 1.103, 1.104), keeping the aortic vent open. The left atrium is then closed.

Right Ventricular Outflow Tract Reconstruction

An appropriate size (26–30 mm) pulmonary homograft previously selected is thawed (if cryopreserved) for 20 minutes. The homograft is checked for any major abnormalities. With interrupted horizontal mattress sutures of 4-0 polypropylene (6–7 in number) the posterior wall of the right ventricular outflow tract is

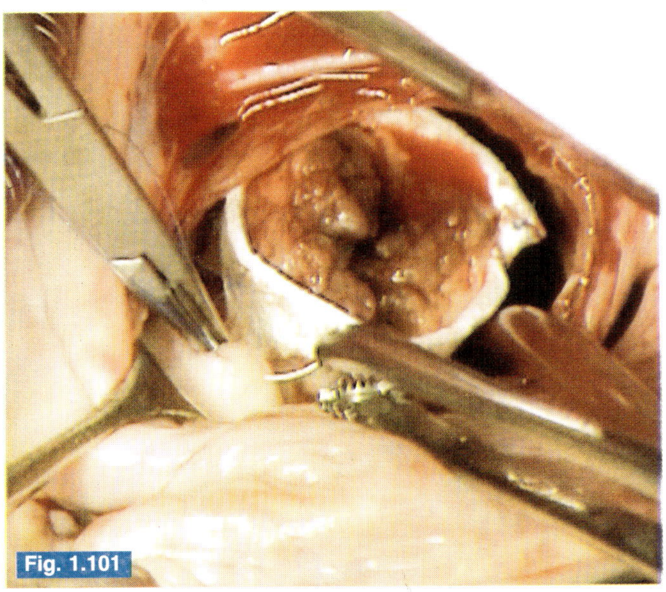

Fig. 1.101

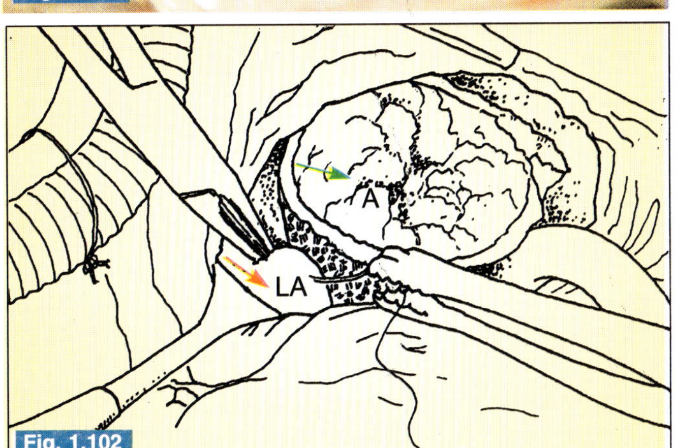

Fig. 1.102

Figs 1.101, 1.102: Suture through left atrial wall (LA) upstream of the annulus. The needle passes through the teflon felt (F) and muscular proximal end of autograft (A). When completed, the teflon felt is buried.

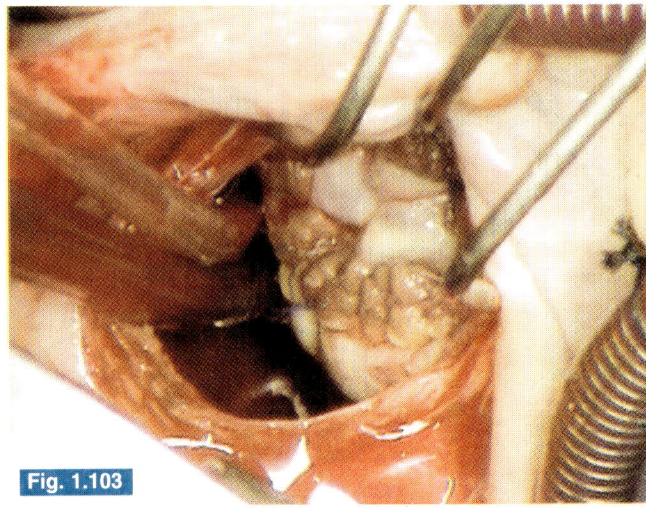

Fig. 1.103

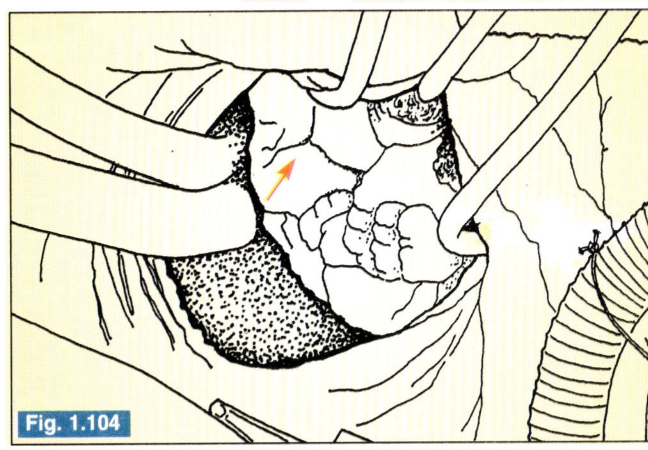

Fig. 1.104

Figs 1.103, 1.104: The pulmonary autograft cusps (arrow) billowing on testing after implantation in the left atrium.

anastomosed to the posterior wall of the homograft (Figs 1.105, 1.106). This suture line is buttressed with a 2–3 mm wide strip of fresh autologous pericardium. When all the sutures are passed the homograft is lowered and the sutures are tied. The first and last sutures on either end are retained and used for continuous anterior anastomosis from either end. Care is exercised to avoid placing the sutures too close to the left main or left anterior descending branch. The anterior suture line is not buttressed with pericardium to avoid gradients by fibrosis (Figs 1.107, 1.108). When the anterior layer is completed, the two ends are tied and cut.

The venous line is partially clamped to fill the right ventricle. This fills the homograft which is closed with the forceps distally. It is checked for leaks and divided at an appropriate length for the distal anastomosis. The clamp on the venous line is removed. All blood in the pericardial cavity is returned via cardiotomy suckers to the oxygenator. The distal pulmonary to pulmonary anastomosis is now begun with a 4-0 polypropylene double arm

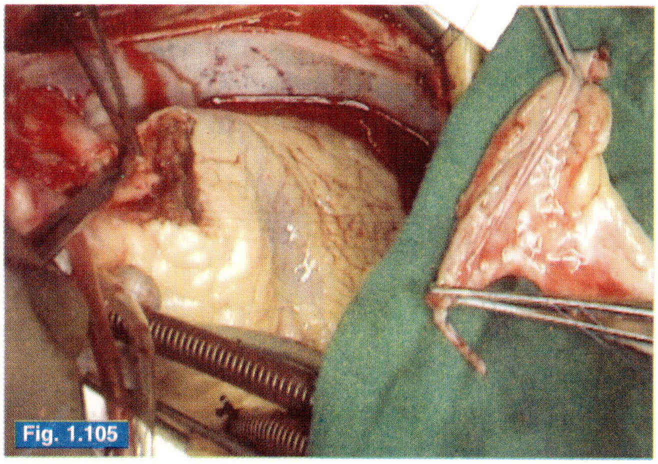

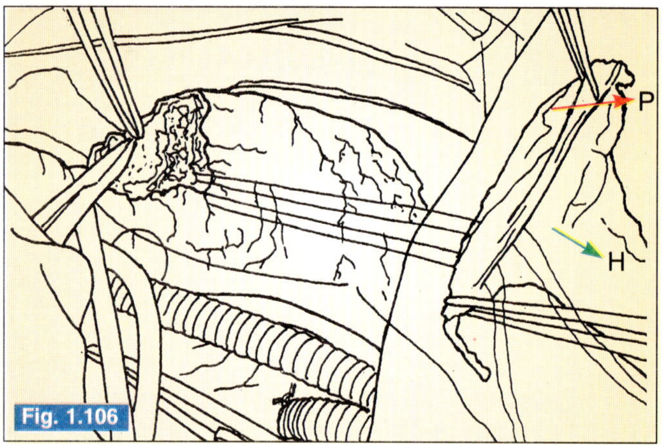

Figs 1.105, 1.106: The interrupted posterior wall anastomoses to the homograft (H) in reconstruction of right ventricular outflow tract. Note pericardial strip (P).

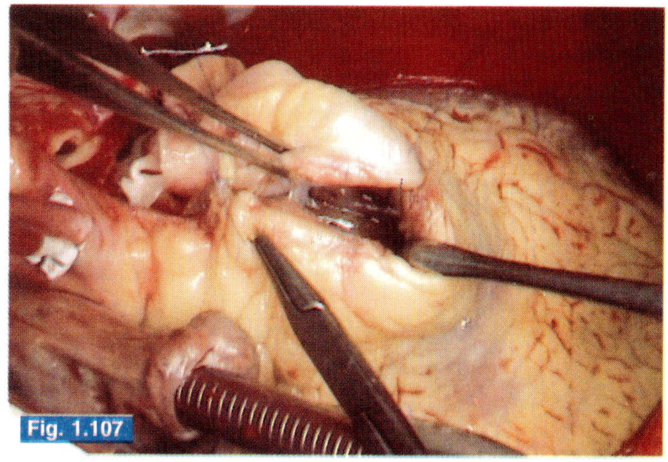

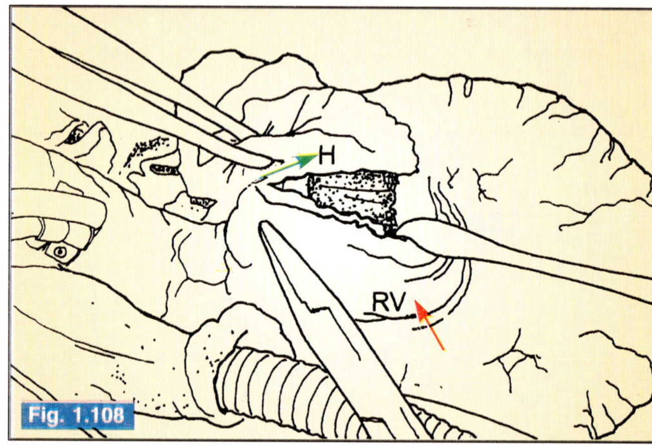

Figs 1.107, 1.108: Reconstruction of the right ventricular outflow tract with a homograft (H); proximal anastomosis to right ventricle (RV).

suture (Figs 1.109, 1.110). The suture begins on the posterior end (6 O'clock position of open pulmonary artery) and comes forward to the 3 O'clock and 9 O'clock positions where it is interrupted to avoid a purse-string effect. It then completes the anterior pulmonary to pulmonary anastomosis. The right ventricle is deaired before completing this suture line. (Figs 1.111–1.112).

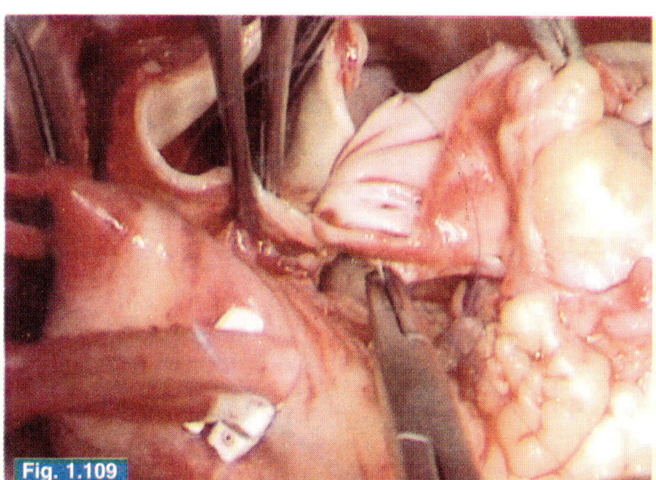

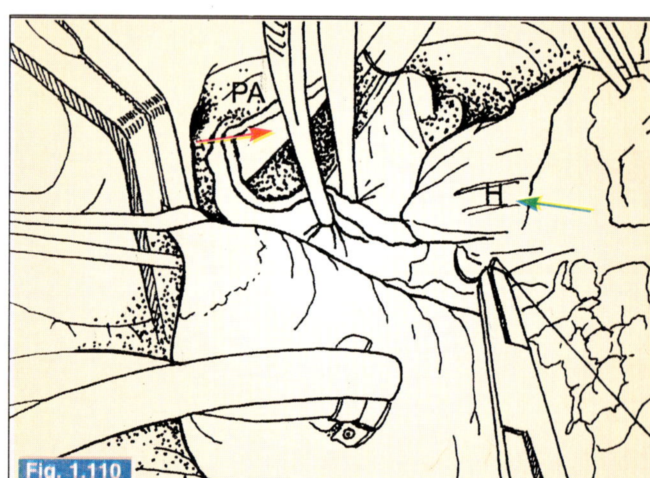

Figs 1.109, 1.110: Pulmonary homograft (H) to pulmonary artery (PA) anastomosis. The first suture for the posterior wall.

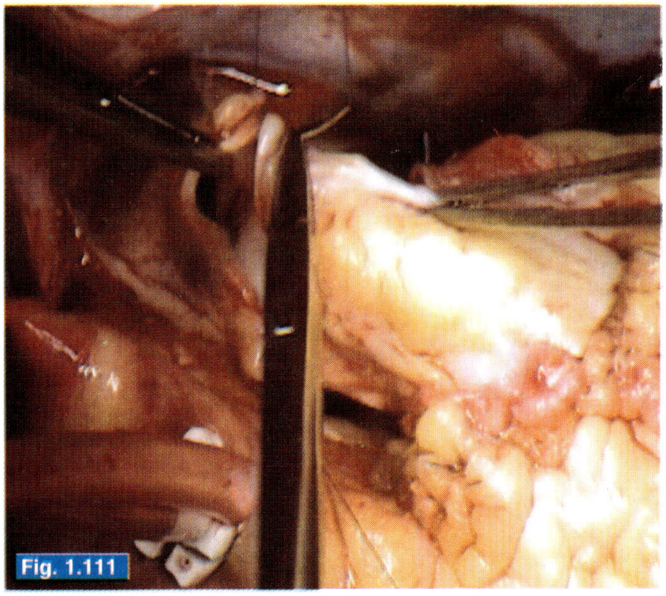

Fig. 1.111

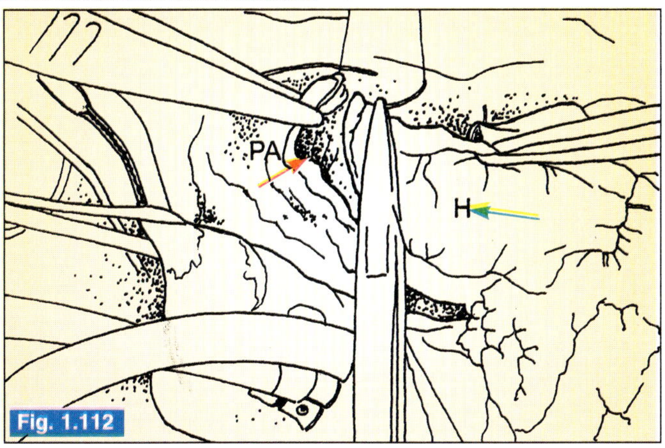

Fig. 1.112

Figs 1.111, 1.112: Pulmonary homograft distal anastomosis to native pulmonary artery, homograft (H), native pulmonary artery (PA). Note thickness of pulmonary artery wall.

Deairing

The left atrial incision is closed after deairing the left atrium. The deairing procedure for bioprosthesis and autograft are similar. Before releasing the aortic clamp the head end is raised. The venous line is partially clamped. The anaesthesiologist is asked to ventilate manually. The aortic root vent is left open to air. The right hand of the surgeon massages the heart. The right index finger and the thumb massage the left atrial appendage and pulmonary veins. When all air is evacuated and there is a continuous flow of blood from the aortic vent, the head end is lowered, cardiopulmonary bypass flow is reduced and the aortic clamp is released. The clamp on the venous line is removed. The head end is raised and aortic vent is placed on strong negative suction (300 ml/min). Gentle massage is continued until the heart begins to beat or is defibrillated.

Postoperative Assessment

This is generally performed by transesophageal echocardiography before heparin reversal. Valve function, presence and severity of paravalvular leaks or mitral regurgitation are noted. This examination should be performed when cardiopulmonary bypass is discontinued and with satisfactory arterial pressure (90 mmHg or more) [Figs 1.113, 1.114].

Complications

Immediate complications include: (a) Bleeding from cardiotomy sites, (b) arrhythmias, and (c) failure to wean from cardiopulmonary bypass. Each one must

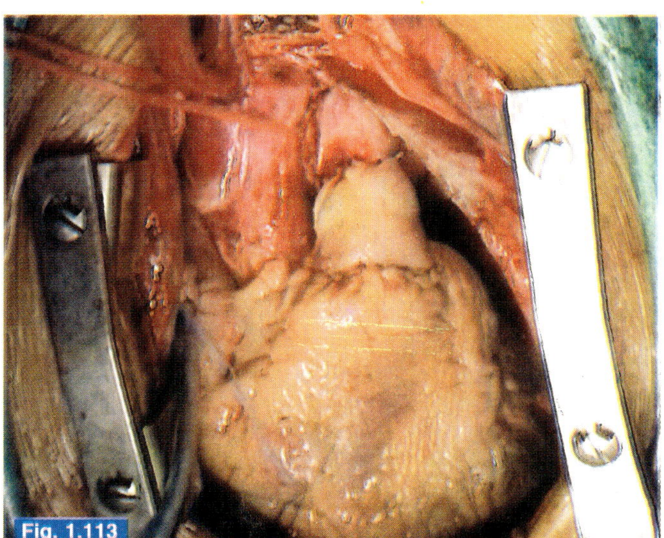

Fig. 1.113

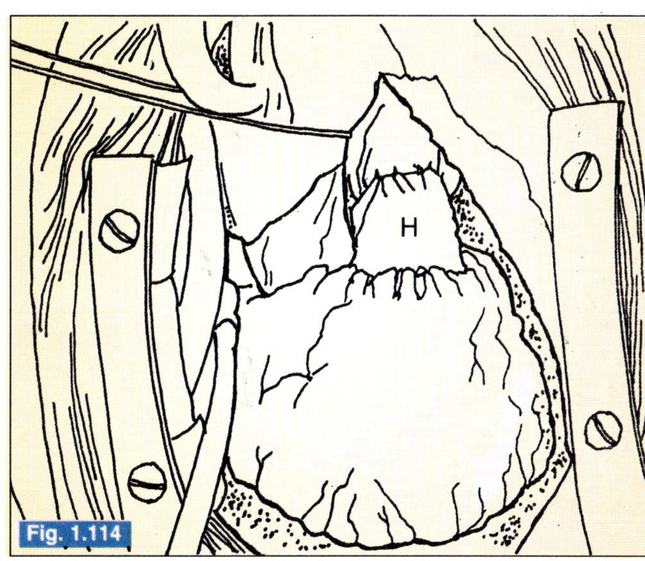

Fig. 1.114

Figs 1.113, 1.114: The heart after completing the Ross-II procedure; pulmonary homograft (H).

be dealt with on its merits. Additional sutures with the heart decompressed usually provide haemostasis.

Correction of hypo/hyperkalaemia, acidosis, generally corrects arrhythmias as also atrial/ ventricular pacing and direct current shock for atrial fibrillation.

Support of the heart in an empty beating state with partial cardiopulmonary bypass and judicious use of inotropes usually corrects the last complication. In open mitral commissurotomy and mitral valve repair inadequate corrections or significant residual mitral regurgitation may require resumption of cardiopulmonary bypass and revision of repair or replacement of the mitral valve.

Early complications include usual general and organ specific complications of cardiopulmonary bypass. A stuck valve can be quickly fatal. It is indicated by a sudden precipitous drop of arterial pressure accompanied by rapid and dangerous rise in left atrial pressure or frank pulmonary oedema. The patient should be returned to the operation theatre, placed on cardiopulmonary bypass and the mitral valve must be rexplored.

Other common early complications seen frequently in any intensive care unit are bleeding, cardiac tamponade, low output syndrome, renal shunt down, arrhythmias, etc. Most resident staff are familiar with the intensive care unit protocols that generally provide adequate guidelines for their management.

Suggested Reading

1 Acar C, Farge A, Ramsheyi A, et al. Mitral valve replacement using a cryopreserved mitral homograft. Ann Thorac Surg 1994;57:746-8.

2 Acar C, Tolan M, Berrebi A, et al. Homograft replacement of the mitral valve: graft selection, technique of implantation, and results in forty-three patients. J Thorac Cardiovasc Surg 1996;111:367-80.

3 Al Hales ZA, Awad MM, Pielers F. Shahid MS. Al Amri MA. Six-year follow up of a pulmonary autograft in the mitral position: the Ross II procedure. J Thorac Cardiovasc Surg 1999;117:614-6.

4 Antunes MJ, Magalhaes MP, Colsen PR, Kinsley RH. Valvuloplasty for rheumatic mitral valve disease. A surgical challenge. J Thorac Cardiovasc Surg 1987;94: 44-56.

5 Becker AE, De Wit AP. Mitral valve apparatus. A spectrum of normality relevant to mitral valve prolapse. Br Heart J. 1979 Dec;42(6):680-9.

6 Carpentier A, Chauvaud S, Fabiani JN, Deloche A, Relland J, Lessana A. Reconstructive surgery of mitral valve in competence: ten-year appraisal. J Thorac Cardiovasc Surg 1980;79:338-48.

7 Choudhary SK, Dhareshwar J, Govil A, Airan B, Kumar AS.Open mitral commissurotomy in the current era : Indications, technique and results. Ann Thorac Surg 2003; 75(1): 41-46.

8 Choudhary SK, Talwar S, Dubey B, Chopra A, Saxena A, Kumar AS. Mitral valve repair in a predominantly rheumatic population : Long term results. Texas Heart Inst J. 2001;28:8-15.

9 Chowdhury UK, Kumar AS, Airan B, Mittal D, Subramaniam KG, Prakash R, Seth S, Singh R, Venugopal P. Mitral valve replacement with and without chordal preservation in a rheumatic population: Serial echocardiographic assessment of left ventricular size and function. Ann Thorac Surg 2005;79:1926-33.

10 Choudhary SK, Talwar S, Juneja R, Kumar AS. Fate of mild aortic valve disease after mitral valve intervention. J Thorac Cardiovasc Surg 2001;122(3):583-6.

11 Cooley DA, Frazier OH, Norman JC. Mitral leaflet prolapse: surgical treatment using a posterior annular collar prosthesis. Cardiovasc Dis, Bull Tex Heart Inst 1976;3:438-43.

12 David TE, Burns RJ, Bacchus CM, Druck MN. Mitral valve replacement for mitral regurgitation with and without preservation of chordae tendineae. J Thorac Cardiovasc Surg 1984;88:718-725.

13 David TE, Uden ED, Strauss HD. The importance of the mitral apparatus in left ventricular function after correction of mitral regurgitation. Circulation 1983;68 (Pt.2): 1176-1182.

14 David TE.Mitral valve replacement with preservation of chordae tendineae: Rationale and technical considerations. Ann Thorac Surg 1986;41:680-682.

15 Deloche A, Jebara VA, Relland JYM, et al. Valve repair with Carpentier techniques. The second decade. J Thorac Cardiovasc Surg 1990;99:990-1002.

16 Di Marco RF, Lee MW, Bekoe S, Grant KJ, Woelfel GF, Pellegrini RV. Interlocking figure of 8 closure of the sternum. Ann Thorac Surg 1989;47(6):927-9.

17 Duran CMG, Gometza B, De Vol EB. Valve repair in rheumatic mitral valve disease. Circulation 1991; 84(Suppl 3):125-32.

18 Eren E, Samilgil A, Ozler A, Ulufer T, Tulpar S. Closed mitral commissurotomy in Istanbul, Turkey: results in 4403 cases. Texas Heart Inst J. 1986 Mar;13(1):143-6.

19 Feikes HL, Daugharthy JB, Perry JE, et al. Preservation of all chordae tendinae and papillary muscle during mitral valve replacement with a tilting disc valve. J Cardiac Surg 1990;5:81-5.

20 Frater RW, Gabbay S, Shore D, Factor S, Strom J. Reproducible replacement of elongated or ruptured mitral valve chordae. Ann Thorac Surg 1983;35:14-28.

21 Gulati GS, Sharma S, Jagia P, Talwar S, Kumar AS. Magnetic resonance imaging of the pulmonary autograft in the mitral position. Texas Heart Inst J. 2004; 31(3):326-7.

22 Hetzer R, Bougioukas G, Franz M, Borst HG. Mitral valve replacement with preservation of papillary muscles and chordae tendineae-revival of a seemingly forgotten concept. Thorac Cardiovasc Surg 1983;31:291-296.

23 Hetzer R, Drews T, Siniawski H, Komoda T, Hofmeister J, Weng Y. Preservation of papillary muscles and chordae during mitral replacement: possibilities and limitations. J Heart Valve Dis 1995;4(Suppl 2): 115-23.

24 Joshi R, Abraham S, Kumar AS. Interlocking sternotomy: Initial experience. Asian Cardiovasc Thorac Ann 2004; 12(1): 16-8.

25 Kabbani SS, Ross DN, Jami H, Hammoud A, Nabhani F. Hariri R, et al. Mitral valve replacement with a pulmonary autograft; initial experience. J Heart Valve Dis. 1999;8:359-67.

26 Kumar AS, Rao PN. Restoration of Pliability to Mitral leaflets during reconstruction. J. Heart Valve Dis. 1995;4:251-253

27 Kumar AS, Kumar DA, Chander H, Saxena A. Experience with Homograft mitral valve replacement. J Heart Valve Dis. 1998;7(2):225-8.

28 KumarAS, Rao PN, Saxena A. Mitral Valve Reconstruction: Eight years experience in 531 patients. J. Heart Valve Dis. 1997;6(6):591-3.

29 Kumar AS, Bhan A, Kumar RV, Shrivastava S, Sood AK, Gopinath N. Cusp-Level Chordal Shortening for Rheumatic Mitral Regurgitation Texas Heart Inst. J 1992, 19(10): 47-50.

30 Kumar AS, Bhan A, Bajaj R, Rao SL, Venugopal P, Shrivastava S. Mitral Valve Repair : Techniques and Results. Ind Heart J.1990;42(3): 135-7.

31 KumarAS, Chander H,Trehan H. Surgical Technique of Multiple Valve replacement with Biological Valves : A New Option. J Heart Valve Dis 1995; 4(1): 45-6.

32 Kumar AS, Agarwal S, Choudhary SK. Mitral valve replacement with pulmonary autograft : Ross II procedure. J Thorac Cardiovasc Surg 2001;122(2): 378-79.

33 Kumar AS, Choudhary SK, Mathur A, Saxena A, Roy R, Chopra P. Homograft mitral valve replacement : Five years' results. J Thorac Cardiovasc Surg 2000;120(3): 450-8.

34 Kumar AS, Dhareshwar J, Airan B, Bhan A, Sharma R,Venugopal P. Redo mitral valve surgery – A long-term experience. J Card Surg 2004 ; 19:303-07.

35 Kumar AS, Kumar RV, Shrivastava S, Venugopal P, Sood AK, Gopinath N. Mitral Valve Reconstruction : Early Results of a Modified Cooley Technique. Texas Heart Inst J. 1992;19(2):107-11.

36 Kumar AS, Prasad S, Rai S, Saxena DK. Right Thoracotomy Revisited. Texas Heart Inst J 1993; 20(1): 40-2.

37 Kumar AS, Rao PN,Saxena DK. Cosmetic Approach to Cardiac Surgery. Asian Cardiovasc and Thorac Annals 1995;3, 20-22.

38 Kumar AS, Rao PN. Mitral Valve Reconstruction : Intermediate Term Results in Rheumatic Mitral Regurgitation. J Heart Valve Dis 1994; 3(2): 161-4.

39 Kumar AS, Trehan H. Homograft Mitral valve replacement : A Case Report. J Heart Valve Dis 1994;3(5):473-5.

40 KumarAS. Rao PN, Saxena A. Results of Mitral valve reconstruction in children with Rheumatic Heart Disease. Ann of Thoracic Surgery 1995; 60(4): 1044-7.

41 Kumar AS. Results of Mitral valve reconstruction in Rheumatic Mitral Regurgitation. Proceedings at 2nd International Conference of Cardiovascular and Thoracic Surgery Puttaparthy. Jan.1994.

42 Kumar AS. Surgery for rheumatic heart disease in Children : Essential Aspects. IAP Journal of Practical Pediatrics 1997; Vol. 5:125-130.

43 Kumar AS. Valvular heart disease - Repair or replacement. J. Ind. Med. Assoc.1999;97:282-86.

44 Lam JH, Ranganathan N, Wigle ED, Silver MD. Morphology of the human mitral valve. I. Chordae tendineae: a new classification. Circulation. 1970 Mar;41(3):449-58.

45 Lillehei CW. New ideas and their acceptance. As it has related to preservation of chordae tendinea and certain other discoveries. J Heart Valve Dis. 1995;4(2):S106-14.

46 Lillehel CW, Levy MJ, Bonnabeau RC Jr. Mitral valve replacement with preservation of papillary muscles and chordae tendineae. J Thorac Cardiovasc Surg 1964;47: 532-543.

47 Miki S, Kusuhara K, Ueda Y, Komeda M, Ohkita Y, Tahata T. Mitral vale replacement with preservation of chordae tendineae and papillary muscles. Ann Thorac Surg. 1988;45(1):28-34.

48 Murala JS, Kumar AS. Long –Term Results of Cusp-Level Chordal Shortening for anterior mitral leaflet prolapse. Texas Heart Inst J 2004;31(3):246-50.

49 Pavankumar P, Venugopal P, Kaul U, Iyer KS, Das B, Airan B, Kumar AS, Rao IM, Sharma ML, Bhatia ML et al. Closed mitral valvotomy during pregnancy. A 20-year experience. Scand.J.Thor.Cardiovasc.Surg.1988;22: 11-15.

50 Reed GE, Kloth HH, Kiely B, Danilowicz DA, Rader B, Doyle EF. Long-term results of mitral annuloplasty in children with rheumatic mitral regurgitation. Circulation. 1974;50(2 Suppl):II189-92.

51 Roy S, Choudhary SK, Kumar AS. Mitral valve repair for nonrheumatic mitral regurgitation. Ind Heart J 2003; 55(4):354-7

52 Silverman ME, Hurst JW. The mitral complex. Interaction of the anatomy, physiology, and pathology of the mitral annulus, mitral valve leaflets, chordae tendineae,

and papillary muscles. Am Heart J. 1968 Sep;76(3):399-418.

53 Talwar S, Mohapatra R, Kumar AS Mitral valve replacement with bioprosthesis : Prevention of suture enlargement. Heart Lung Circ. 2006 Feb;15(1):48-9.

54 Talwar S, Rajesh MR, Subramanian A, Saxena A, Kumar AS. Mitral valve repair in children with rheumatic heart disease. J Thorac Cardiovasc Surg 2005; 129(4):875-9.

55 Van Rijk-Zwikker GL, Delemarre BJ, Huysmans HA. Mitral valve anatomy and morphology: relevance to mitral valve replacement and valve reconstruction. J. Card Surg. 1994 Mar;9(2 Suppl):255-61.

56 Victor S, Nayak VM. Skirts, slits, scallops and semantics. J Heart Valve Dis. 1995; 4: 576-79.

57 Wasir H, Choudhary SK, Airan B, Srivastava S, Kumar AS. Mitral Valve Replacement with chordal preservation in a Rheumatic Population. J Heart Valve Dis 2001;10(1): 84-9.

58 Yacoub MH, Kittle CF. A new technique for replacement of the mitral valve by a semilunar valve homograft. J. Thorac Cardiovasc Surg. 1969;58:859-69.

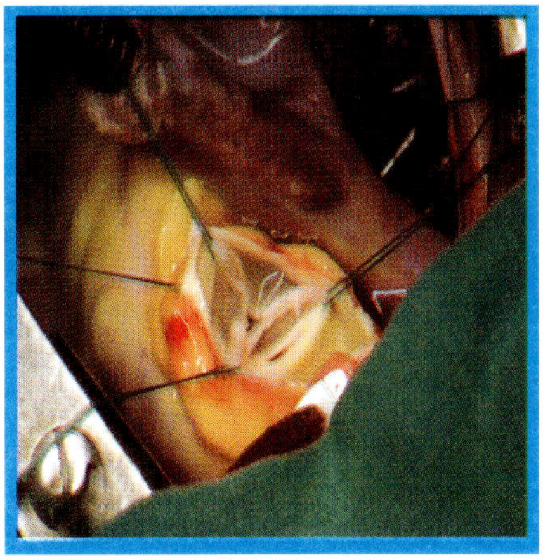

2 The Aortic Valve

Anatomy

The human aortic valve is wedged between the tricuspid/ mitral and pulmonary valves. It is usually tricuspid and has close relationships to anterior mitral leaflet, atrioventricular node and bundle of His, and to the coronary arteries. For a complete description of the anatomy, the reader may refer to the publications given at the end of this chapter.

Physiology

The aortic and pulmonary valves are derived from the truncal valve and are identical in structure and function. They can, therefore, be used for substitution when required.

The sinuses of the aortic valve are essential for its normal function, especially for its competence. Function of the aortic valve is best studied in the intact patient by transesophageal echocardiography. With a short axis cross-sectional view, morphology and function can be studied. In a long axis view stenosis, regurgitation and abnormalities of the subaortic region can be clearly visualised.

It is interesting to note that the normal aortic valve opens only partially in the resting, anaesthetised patient but opens fully as the stroke volume increases. A rigid mitral ring / prosthesis usually creates a gradient in the left ventricular outflow tract. Similarly some chordal preservation techniques (when not performed well) and struts of a bioprosthesis (when improperly oriented) may cause significant left ventricular outflow tract gradients. The normal (mean) human aortic valve diameter is 23.3 mm in adult males and 21.6 mm in the adult female.

Pathology

Aortic valve disease in the young may be due to congenital abnormalities. Common among these is congenital aortic stenosis and bicuspid aortic valve with aortic stenosis/aortic regurgitation.

It may be due to rheumatic heart disease in which aortic regurgitation is usually predominant but may be combined with aortic stenosis. However, pure aortic stenosis in rheumatic heart disease is extremely rare. In older patients it is common and is considered degenerative (an aging process) as seen in Fig. 2.1. Calcification is quite common in the elderly and may be associated with atherosclerosis.

Infective endocarditis is one of the common causes of severe aortic regurgitation and usually affects a diseased or deformed valve.

Traumatic rupture and aortic dissection complete the rare causes of aortic regurgitation.

Selection of Procedure

In order to select an appropriate procedure for a patient with aortic valve disease, age, aetiology and aortic annulus diameter are considered. Appendix I provides guidelines for selection. It is presumed, however, that a tissue valve bank or access to homografts is freely available before making the selection.

AORTIC STENOSIS

Valvular aortic stenosis is almost always congenital in origin. The cusps are usually fused and produce severe gradients in infants and children. Diagnosis is easily established with echocardiography.

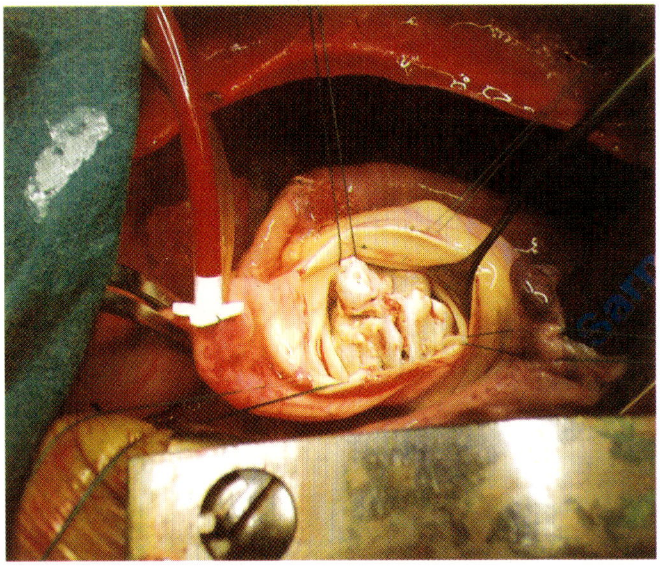

Fig. 2.1: Calcific aortic stenosis.

The treatment of choice is aortic valve balloon dilatation which can be life saving at times. This procedure is preferred over open commissurotomy. Also, it provides an opportunity for growth of the annulus with somatic growth so that a more definitive operation can be postponed to a slightly older age (childhood/adolescence). However, it may produce significant aortic regurgitation which can be controlled with medical management.

Open commissurotomy introduces the risk of cardiopulmonary bypass, and reoperation. However, at open commissurotomy other problems such as a subvalvular or supravalvular obstruction can be relieved. Valve replacement in such young patients is best avoided. When aortic valve replacement is mandatory, the pulmonary autograft (Ross procedure) is the best substitute.

Surgical Technique

Aortic Valvotomy

For isolated aortic valve surgery, the cardiopulmonary bypass may be slightly modified. Generally a single cannula in the right atrium is sufficient for adequate venous drainage. The aortic cannula is placed as high on the ascending aorta as possible. Two stay sutures are placed on the ascending aorta about 4–5 mm distal to the right coronary artery origin (Figs 2.2, 2.3). The cardioplegia cannula (also used as aortic vent) should be placed as far away from the aortotomy site, with sufficient length for clamping between it and the aortic cannula.

A vent is placed through the right superior pulmonary vein left atrial junction. This is done as soon as the aorta is clamped. Normothermic perfusion is preferred. The aortic incision is transverse at first and after placing the vent and emptying the heart and aorta, under vision the incision is extended to the left side. Here it is curved upwards so that the pulmonary artery is not injured. On the right side the aortotomy extends down into the middle of the noncoronary sinus, but stops short of the annulus by at least 5 mm. Cardioplegia is usually delivered into the aortic root if there is no aortic regurgitation. If aortic regurgitation is present then it should delivered directly into the coronary ostia. Flexible, graduated coronary perfusion cannulae are commercially available for this purpose. Topical ice slush is used for myocardial cooling.

On completion of cardioplegia infusion the vent is placed on negative suction and all excess fluid and ice water and discarded through the waste suction line.

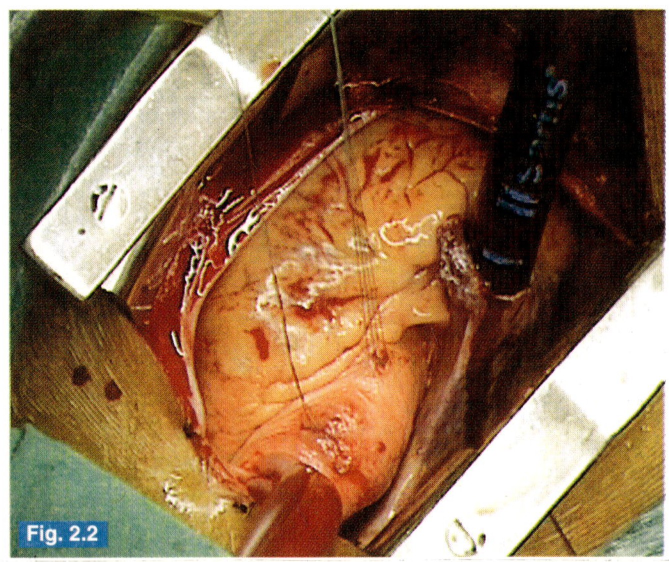

Fig. 2.2

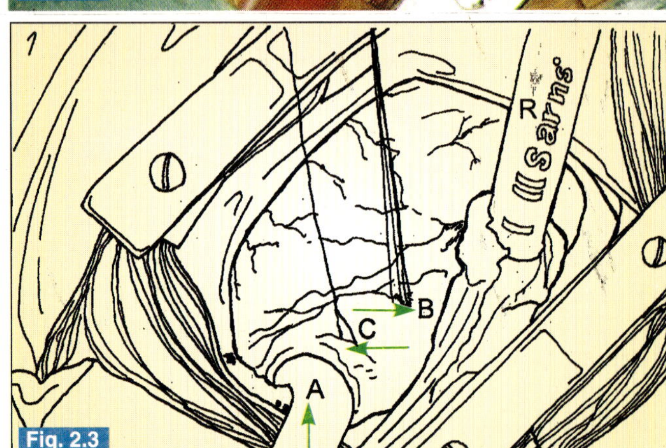

Fig. 2.3

Figs 2.2, 2.3: Location of aortic (A) and right atrial (R) cannulae. Note sites for aortotomy (B) and cardioplegia cannula (C).

The aortic valve is best exposed by three commissural stay sutures placed at the top of each commissure. These are pulled up and clipped to the drapes with haemostats. This delivers the aortic valve into the aortotomy incision. The valve is now inspected and its morphology noted.

With the tip of a no. 11 blade the commissures are divided in an outward direction from the aortic valve orifice. Care and patience are essential ingredients for a successful valvotomy. The assistant retracts the cusps as the incision is extended towards commissure. This procedure is used to split the other two commissures as well. Following commissural incision the subvalvular left ventricular outflow tract is inspected. The thickened endocardium that is almost always found here is gently grasped with a tissue forceps and peeled downwards towards the left ventricular cavity. This procedure may also be required to remove the endocardial peel from the anterior mitral leaflet as well. Extreme care and gentle handling will provide the best results. With a thin ribbon retractor placed into the aortic valve orifice the right coronary cusps is retracted and held by the assistant. The interior of the left ventricle is carefully inspected for endocardial thickening, discrete membrane, etc. When satisfied, a graduated Hegar dilator is passed. The largest size of the dilator that can be passed without difficulty is noted. Care must be taken not to injure the aortic cusps at this stage.

The aortotomy incision is now closed with 5-0 prolene running suture. The left ventricular vent is clamped and the patient is rewarmed.

Deairing

The venous return tubing is partially clamped. The left atrial vent is clamped. The aortic vent is opened to air. With the right hand the heart is gently massaged, inverting the left atrial appendage, squeezing the pulmonary veins etc. until there is a continuous flow of blood in the aortic vent. The anaesthesiologist gently ventilates the patient at this time. When satisfied the head end is lowered and aortic clamp is released slowly. The aortic vent is placed on strong negative suction (300 ml/min). The left atrial vent is released and the clamp on the venous line is removed. The heart is gently massaged. If spontaneous sinus rhythm resumes, partial bypass is continued. If the heart fibrillates, it is defibrillated with a direct current shock. At this time it is good to observe the heart for any left ventricular dysfunction (residual aortic regurgitation), rhythm (heart block?) and palpate the aorta for any thrill when ejections begin. When all is satisfactory, left atrial vent is removed and the site oversewn. Aortotomy is inspected for leaks. Cardiopulmonary bypass is discontinued slowly when the ejections are satisfactory. A systolic aortic pressure of 50–60 mm is acceptable at this stage. The aortic vent remains on strong suction for at least 5 min after cardiopulmonary bypass is discontinued.

A transesophageal echocardiography confirms satisfactory vatrotomy and reduction of gradients. Mild aortic regurgitation is acceptable and one should not be too enthusiastic to obtain a perfect result. A gradient of 10–20 mm (from 90–100 mm Hg) can be accepted. Haemostasis and chest closure follow. The pericardium must be closed with interrupted sutures for a safe re-entry at the next surgery.

Results

Early results are extremely gratifying. If performed in time, valvular aortic stenosis can be corrected without mortality. Risk factors for mortality include additional cardiac anomalies like ventricular septal defect, coarctation, tunnel left ventricular outflow tract obstruction and gross congestive heart failure. Patients should be followed up at six-monthly intervals for gradient, progression of aortic regurgitation and left ventricular function, by echocardiography. Reoperation rates are high and almost all patients will require valve replacement by 10 years. However, the operation provides an opportunity for somatic growth and better surgical options in older children.

Aortic stenosis in adults is indeed a completely different problem. In younger patients (adolescents and adults) the cause is almost always congenital, especially a bicuspid aortic valve. Many of these patients may have undergone a previous aortic valve baloon dilatation or surgical valvotomy. In older patients degenerative aortic valve disease causes severe calcific aortic stenosis (Fig. 2.1). Mild degrees of aortic regurgitation may be present when the aortic valve is rigid and immobile with a fixed orifice. Diagnosis is established by echocardiography. Surgery is generally recommended if the gradient is 50 mm or more or the patient presents with symptoms such as syncope, angina, etc. Sudden death from arrhythmias is a serious risk. Long standing aortic stenosis may produce severe left ventricular dysfunction with pulmonary hypertension. It is preferable to offer surgery before left ventricular dysfunction sets in. An aortic root injection, left ventricular injection and selective coronary angiography should be performed in patients over the age of 40 years to exclude significant coronary artery disease.

Transoesophageal Echocardiography

Transoesophageal echocardiography is performed soon after the patient is intubated. Generally two or three views are sufficient for a complete analysis—four-chamber view, a short axis view of the aortic valve and a long axis view. It is important to assess the mitral valve carefully for thickening (jet lesion), mitral regurgitation, etc. Aortic valve morphology, annulus diameter, calcification and pulmonary valve morphology and diameter are assessed. It is important for the surgeon to learn to perform transesophageal echocardiography himself as explained earlier.

AORTIC VALVE REPLACEMENT

Surgical Approach

Approach is best through a midsternotomy incision. A single two-stage venous cannula and aortic cannulation are performed for cardiopulmonary bypass. Stay sutures are placed 1 cm distal to right coronary artery ostium. An aortic vent cannula is placed on the highest point of ascending aorta. Normothermic perfusion is used. Left atrial vent is placed through right superior pulmonary vein.

Myocardial protection requires special attention in aortic stenosis because of ventricular hypertrophy. Cold hyperkalaemic blood cardioplegia is injected directly into the left coronary artery and right coronary artery after aortotomy. Topical ice slush is used for myocardial cooling. Cardioplegia is repeated every 20 minutes.

Historically continuous coronary perfusion, retrograde coronary sinus cardioplegia and continuous topical hypothermia have been used successfully. However the distribution of cardioplegic solution, complete electromechanical arrest and smooth post surgical recovery are best with antegrade cardioplegia. In addition intermittent cardioplegic injection provides the best operating conditions for aortic valve replacement, especially in the small aortic root.

Choice of Valve Substitute

To decide the most appropriate option for aortic valve replacement, three variable are considered: (1) Aortic annulus diameter, (2) etiology, and (3) age of the patient (see Appendix I).

If the aortic annulus measures 30 mm or more, a mechanical valve is the best option in all patients up to the age of 50 years.

If the aortic annulus measures less than 30 mm, other options based on etiology and age are considered. For patients with rheumatic heart disease who are young (less than 35 years), a homograft aortic valve replacement by the scallopped subcoronary technique is the best option since they are likely to return for reoperation in 15–20 years. If a homograft is not available, a mechanical valve is the next best option.

If the patient is between 35 and 50 years (rheumatic heart disease), a Ross procedure is the operation of choice. In the absence of facilities for a valve bank, a mechanical valve is the next best alternative.

In patients with congenital heart disease (bicuspid aortic valve), a Ross procedure is the operation of choice from neonates to 50 years of age.

For patients over the age of 50 years with rheumatic, congenital or degenerative aortic valve disease, the substitute of choice is a tissue valve. Currently available tissue valves (pericardial) are expected to last for nearly 20 years.

Aortic Valve Replacement with Mechanical Valve

An oblique aortotomy incision is used as described earlier for aortic valvotomy. After cardioplegia delivery the cannula remains in the left coronary artery ostium preventing calcific and other debris from entering the left coronary artery.

The 2-0 braided stay sutures are taken at the top of the commissures and pulled up to the drapes (Figs 2.4, 2.5). This manoeuvre delivers the aortic valve into the aortotomy incision. The valve cusps are excised taking care to avoid injury to the anterior mitral leaflet. When calcified, it is best to remove the valve partially at first and under vision complete the excision (Figs 2.6, 2.7). A small wet sponge is placed just below the valve in the left ventricular outflow tract, to prevent calcific debris falling into the left ventricle. The valve remnants are excised with care using the tip of a No. 11 blade. A right-angled clamp may be used just below the commissures to coax fibrous and calcific nodules to separate from the endocardium. Calcium is removed with meticulous care especially when it extends into the interventricular septum or anterior mitral leaflet. Thickened and fibrous endocardial peel should be removed from the left ventricular outflow tract. This prevents development of subvalvular gradients postoperatively and also permits implantation of a larger size valve. If aortic regurgitation is present the anterior mitral leaflet is usually thickened and

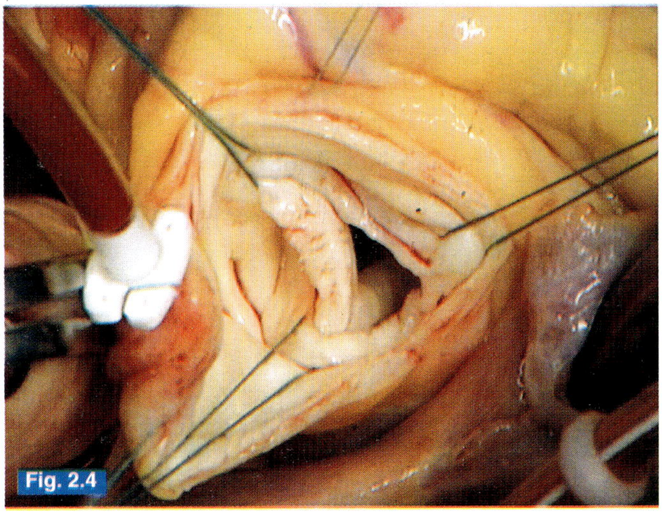
Fig. 2.4

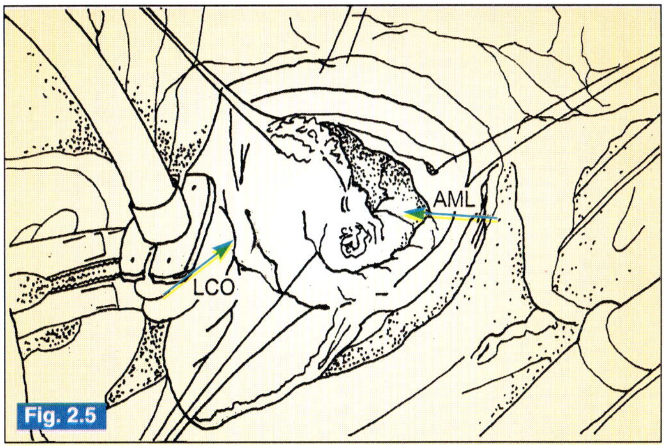

Fig. 2.5

Figs 2.4, 2.5: The three stay sutures at the top of the commissural pillars that deliver the aortic valve into the aortotomy; left coronary ostium (LCO), anterior mitral leaflet (AML).

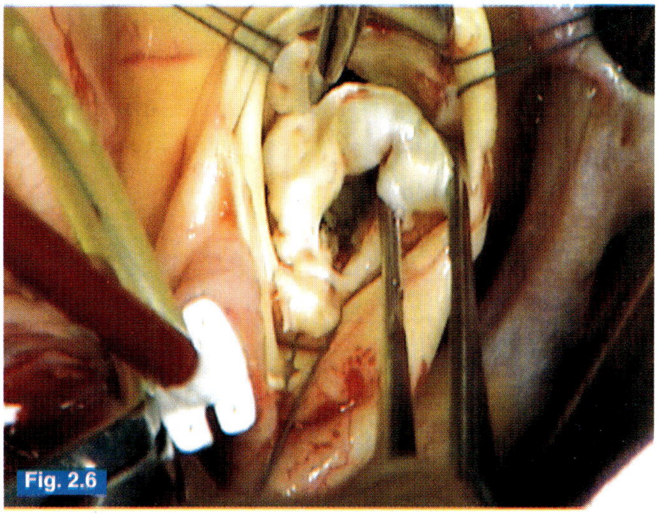
Fig. 2.6

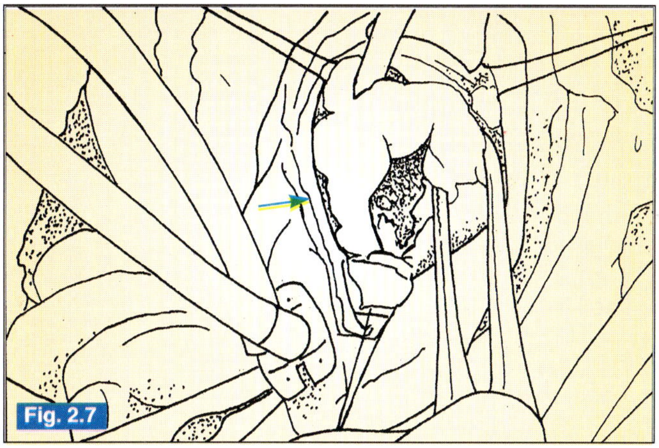
Fig. 2.7

Figs 2.6, 2.7: Excision of a calcific aortic valve. Note left coronary

peels easily. The aortic annulus is palpated for any residual calcium. When excision is completed, the sponge in the left ventricular outflow tract is removed. The left ventricular vent is put off. The left ventricular cavity and the ascending aorta proximal to the aortic clamp are washed vigorously several times with ice cold solution and discarded through the waste suction. The coronary cannula in the left coronary artery ostium is left in place during the washing.

The aortic annulus is measured with the standard valve sizers (Fig. 2.8). It is not unusual to find a larger annulus following excision of calcific and stenotic valve than was measured by transesophageal echocardiography. In rheumatic heart disease the annulus sometimes measures more than 30 mm.

An appropriate size valve is selected. It is necessary to orient the valve before hand if it is non rotatable. The assistant holds to valve holder towards the head end of the aortotomy. Simple, single,

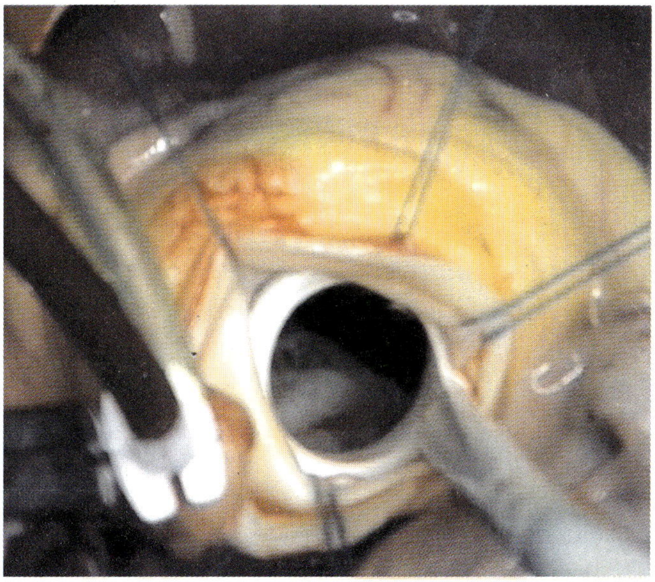

Fig. 2.8: Sizing the aortic annulus. The sizer is rotated at the annulus and moved in and out of the left ventricle to decide the appropriate size.

interrupted sutures of 2-0 braided are passed through the aortic annulus exiting on the left ventricular side. The needle is then passed through the sewing rim of the prosthesis. The right coronary sinus sutures are taken first (Fig. 2.9). Usually 6–8 sutures are placed irrespective of the valve size. Pledgeted sutures are not required for routine valve replacement. In the author's experience (more than 2000 aortic valve replacement) pledgeted sutures were used only very rarely to fit a smaller valve in a hugely dilated aortic annulus (Marfan's) or when the aortic annulus is friable. The left coronary and noncoronary sutures are placed in that order (Figs 2.10, 2.11). Each is held on a haemostat. The aortic commissural stay sutures are removed. The valve is lowered with care to avoid entanglement of sutures. The three commissural sutures are tied first to ensure proper seating of the valve. It is preferable to use alternating colours (green/white/blue) for ease of identification and for tying. Care must be taken to seat the valve properly in the annulus especially at the struts which must lie in the left ventricle and not in the aortic sinus. Once all sutures are tied the valve is rotated and oriented where the disc/discs are freely mobile without obstruction (Figs 2.12, 2.13). For tilting disc valves the larger orifice is best oriented towards to the noncoronary sinus (Fig. 2.14). The coronary ostia are also inspected for obstruction.

The aortotomy is now closed with two 4-0 polypropylene sutures while the left ventricular vent is clamped and patient is rewarmed. A 2 layer suture line ensures proper haemostasis.

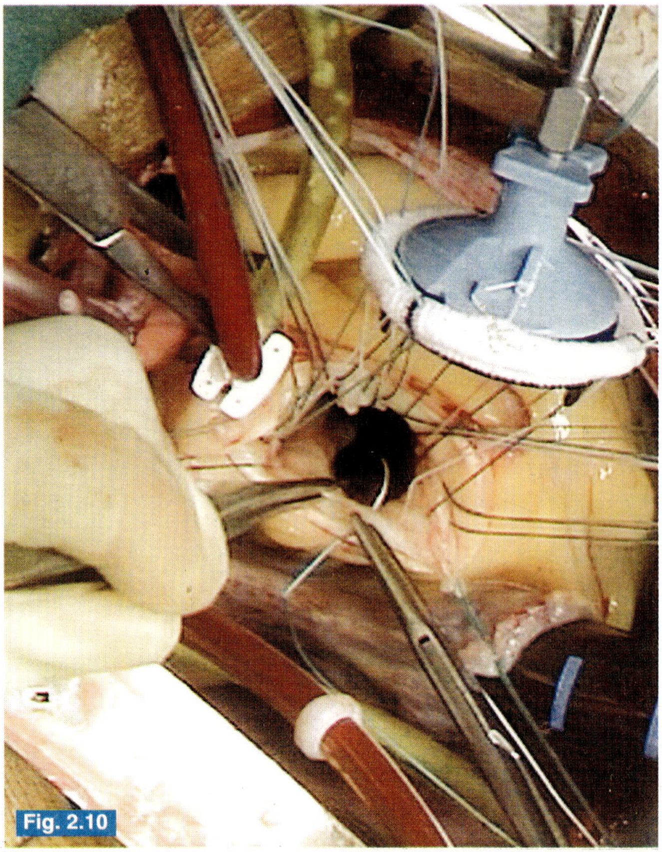

Fig. 2.10

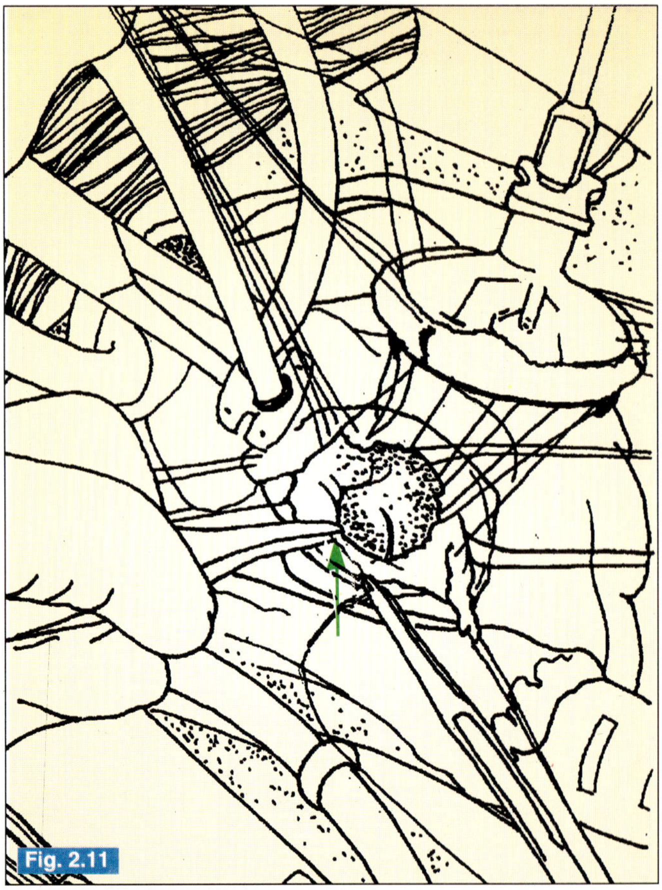

Fig. 2.11

Figs 2.10, 2.11: Backhand sutures for the annulus below the non coronary sinus (arrow).

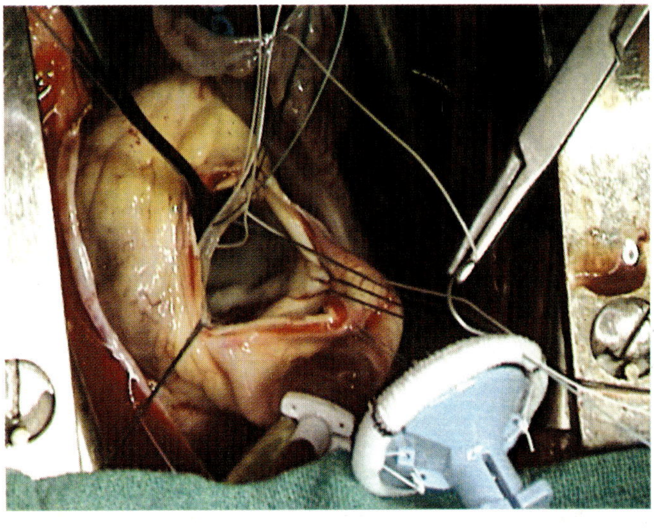

Fig. 2.9: Implantation of a mechanical valve. Note how a forehand suture picks up the annulus below the right coronary sinus and the needle passes forehand again through the sewing cuff.

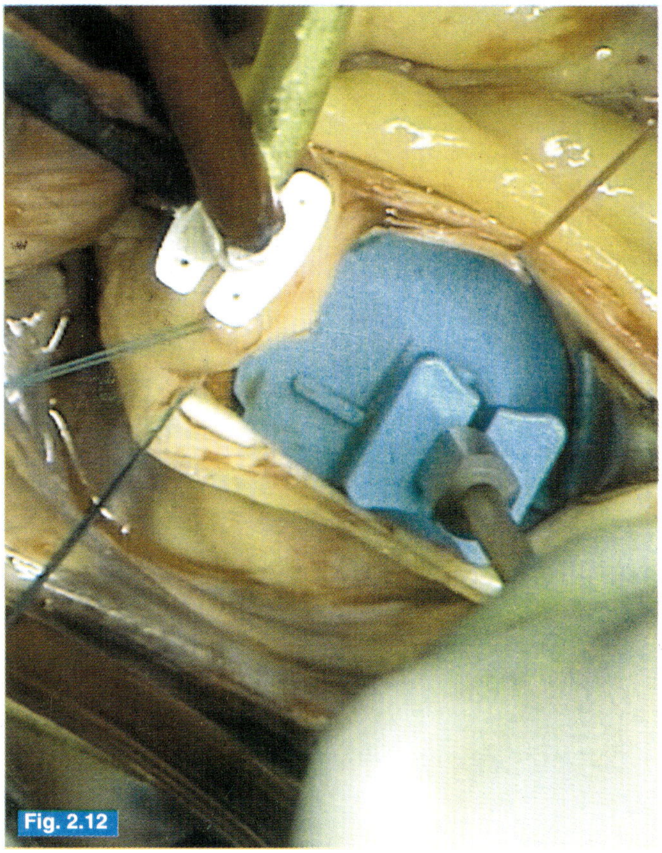

Fig. 2.12

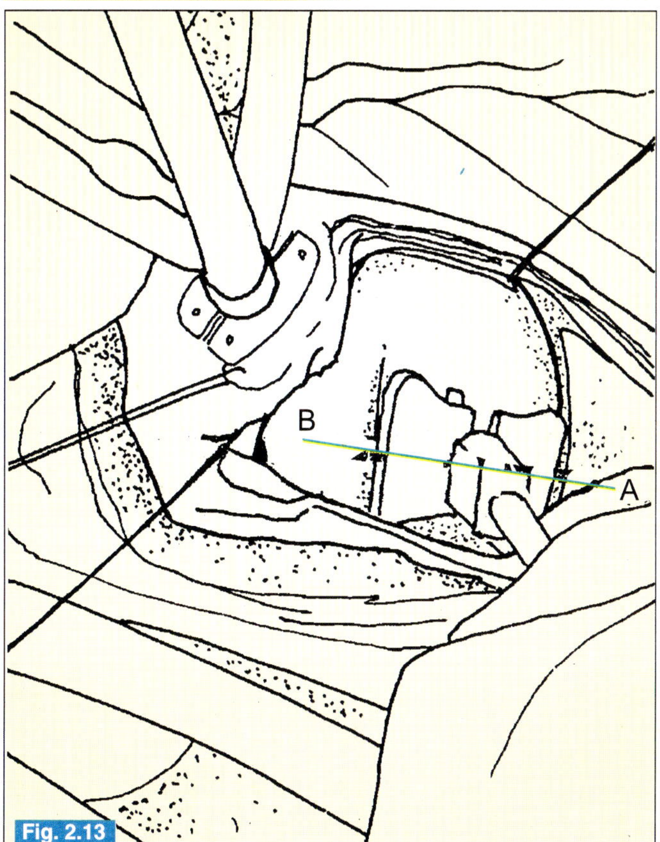

Fig. 2.13

Figs 2.12, 2.13: Rotation of the mechanical valve after implantation. The rotator handle (A–B) is at a right angle to the hingeline of the discs.

Deairing

When the patient temp is 36°C or higher (37°C) the venous drainage line is partially clamped. The left atrial vent remains clamped. The heart is gently massaged and air is evacuated through the aorta while the anaesthetist ventilates the lungs. When satisfied the head end is lowered and the aortic clamp is removed slowly allowing the aortic vent to bleed freely. The aortic vent is then put on negative suction (300 ml/min). The venous line clamp is removed and left atrial vent is placed on gentle suction. The right hand continues to massage the heart gently until it resumes beating or is defibrillated. In hypertrophied hearts it may take a few minutes before spontaneous heartbeat begins. When small ejections become apparent the left atrial vent is clamped and removed. The heart is supported with partial cardiopulmonary bypass until satisfactory cardiac action is evident. When satisfactory, cardiopulmonary bypass is gradually discontinued. The aortic vent is placed on strong suction for another 5 minutes. A systolic aortic pressure of 70–80 mm of Hg is accepted with a small dose (0.25 mg /kg) nitroglycerine infusion begun when rewarming. Patients with severe aortic stenosis and hypertrophied hearts require higher filling pressures (right atrium of 6–10 mm Hg) for satisfactory haemodynamics. If there is slow nodal rhythm or heart block is present, ventricular pacing is begun before

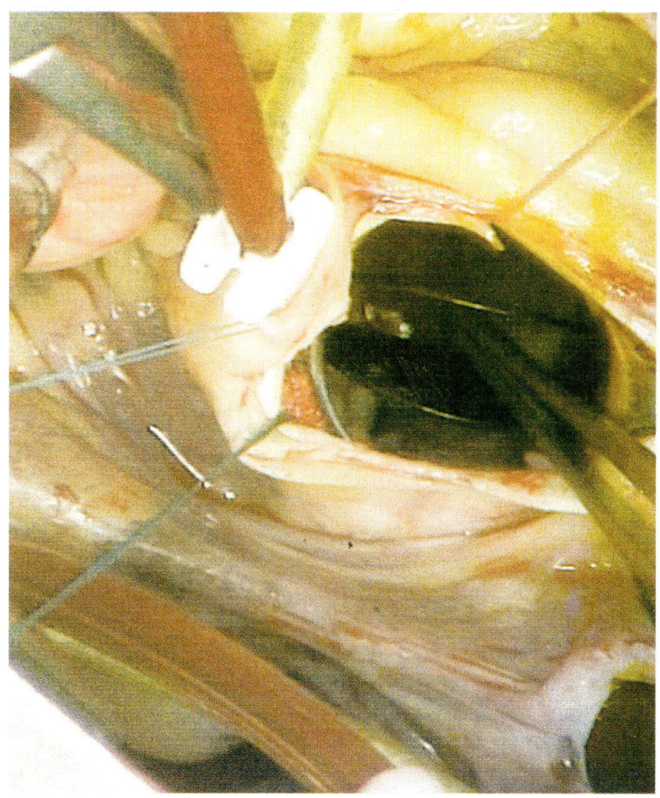

Fig. 2.14: The completed implantation, ensuring free movement of discs.

discontinuing cardiopulmonary bypass. In the author's experience inotropic support (Dopamine/ Dobutamine) are almost never required in these powerful hearts. With stable haemodynamics, decannulation and heparin reversal can be done.

Results

Aortic valve replacement with mechanical valve is a universally performed operation. Almost every qualified cardiac surgeon has performed aortic valve replacement. Over the past 3 decades in over 4000 patients (operated in our institution) our experience has demonstrated a falling operative mortality. For isolated aortic valve replacement currently the operative mortality is 0%. Risk factors for mortality include presence of coronary artery disease, higher age (>75 yr), chronic obstructive pulmonary disease, obesity and poor left ventricular function. An effort should be made to implant a large valve in each case. In the author's experience 75% of patients undergoing isolated aortic valve replacement receive a valve 25 mm or higher even in patients with aortic stenosis. It is not unusual to see 29 and 31 mm (and rarely 33 mm) valves being implanted. Postoperative gradients will be negligible and exercise tolerance will be better.

Aortic Valve Replacement with Tissue Valves

There are few if any differences in the technique of implantation of a tissue valves as compared to a mechanical valve.

Choice of Tissue Valve

Stented *vs.* Stentless

Stented Tissue Valve Implantation

In measuring the size of valve to use, apart from the aortic annulus diameter, some manufacturer's recommend measuring the sinotubular junction diameter as well.

The stent posts must be oriented properly so that they do not obstruct the coronaries. The valve cannot be rotated and so proper orientation before placing the sutures is vital (Figs 2.15, 2.16). When tying the sutures care must be taken to push the tissue valve sewing ring down to the aortic annulus. In addition distortion of stent posts must be avoided during tying of the knots (Figs 2.17, 2.18, 2.19).

The tissue valves are usually stored in gluteraldehyde and they must be rinsed thoroughly for

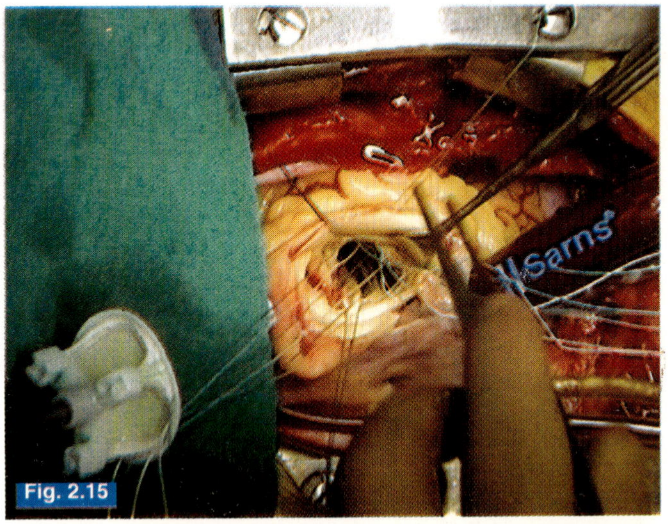

Fig. 2.15

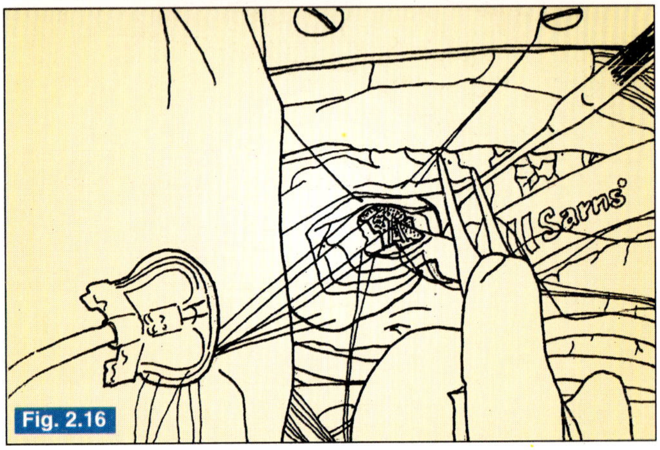

Fig. 2.16

Figs 2.15, 2.16: Technique of suturing single; simple sutures without pledges.

3 min each in two bowls of saline and during implantation the cusps must be moistened frequently to prevent their drying.

Stentless Tissue Valve

At present there are several different stentless valves available for aortic valve replacement. All are porcine valves.

The stentless valves have circular sewing cuff like the mechanical valve. In addition they also have commissural posts that need fixing. Again orientation of these valves must be decided before hand so that coronary ostial obstruction is avoided. The proximal suture line is usually with interrupted 4-0 braided suture. The distal suture line for the commissural posts is usually 15–20 mm from the annulus and corresponds to the top of the aortic sinuses. The stentless valves need to be anchored like the homograft in the scalloped subcoronary technique, which will be described with implantation of the

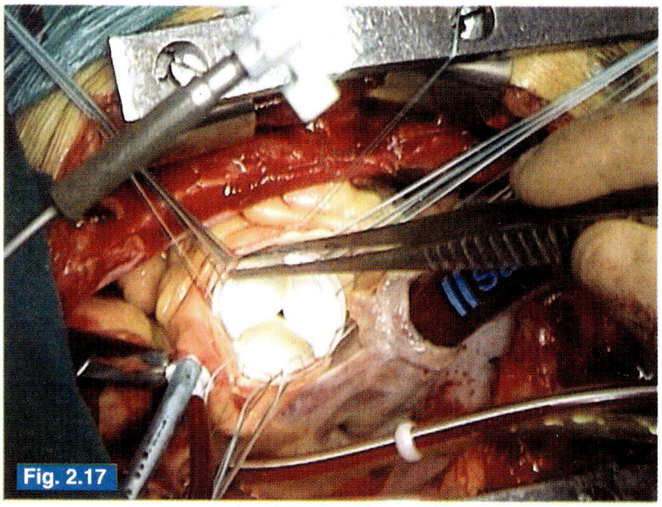

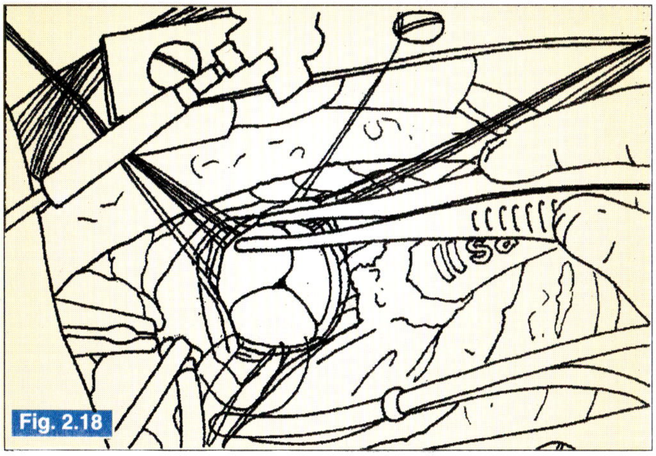

Figs 2.17, 2.18: Seating of the tissue valve in the aortic position.

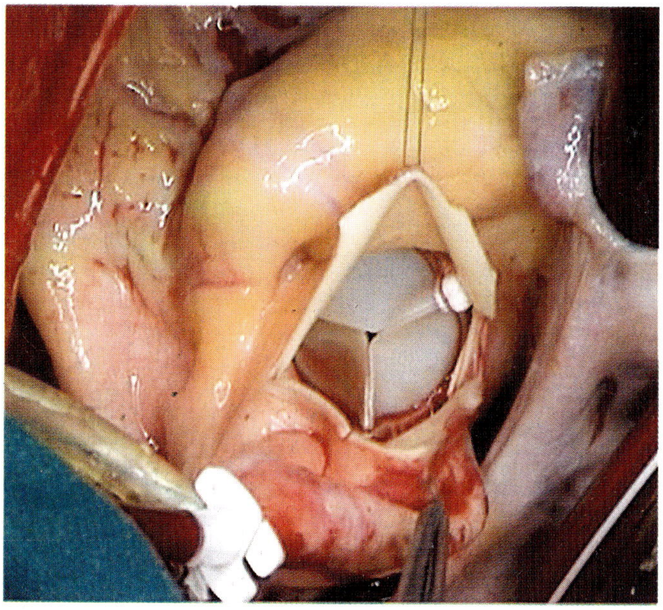

Fig. 2.19: The completed operation. Note location of struts in relation to the coronary ostia and aortotomy incision.

homograft. They may also be implanted as a full root. This technique is described under ROSS procedure.

Stentless valves provide a larger effective orifice and better haemodynamics, less gradients compared to the stented valves. However, they are more expensive and do not have any additional advantage in durability.

Aortic Valve Replacement with a Homograft

As described earlier, the choice of a substitute depends on aortic annuls diameter, aetiology and age. A root diameter less than 30 and young (less than 35) patient with rheumatic heart disease is the ideal candidate (Figs 2.20, 2.21). The decision to use a homograft is made on transesophageal echocardiography and is subject to ready availability of an appropriate sized homograft. A scalloped subcoronary technique is preferable in the young rheumatic heart disease patient because they will certainly require a second operation. This permits near normal external anatomy for a safe second operation.

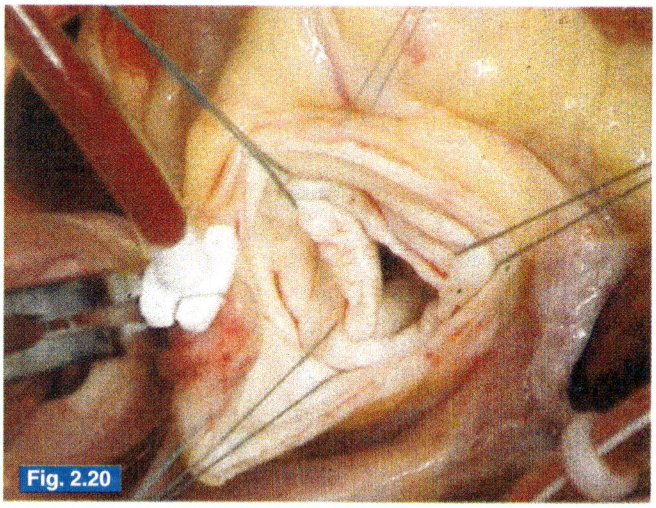

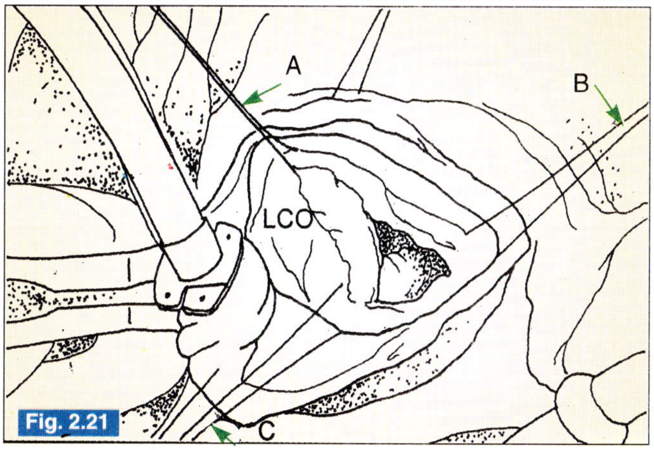

Figs 2.20, 2.21: Fibrosed aortic valve. The three commissural sutures (A, B and C) and the left coronary ostium (LCO).

The root replacement technique although considered the ideal technique is best used in older patients and for infective endocarditis where there is considerable destruction of tissue with abscesses and even discontinuity from left ventricle to aorta. This technique is especially useful for prosthetic valve endocarditis where it may be life saving.

Scalloped Subcoronary Implantation

An aortic homograft (fresh or cryopreserved) whose diameter is 2–3 mm less than the aortic annulus diameter is chosen. If cryopreserved, thawing should begin with the skin incision since it may take nearly 30 min to thaw (see valve banking for thawing protocol). If fresh antibiotic preserved, it can be used immediately without further processing. Pulmonary homografts are not suitable for aortic valve replacement.

Preparation for Implantation

The homograft is trimmed of muscle, tissue and fat. The coronary ostia are identified. It is inspected for any damage to the cusps during harvesting. Distally it is cut across 3–4 mm above the top of the commissural pillars (Figs 2.22, 2.23). All the three sinuses may be excised leaving a 3–4 mm aortic wall at the base of the sinus and all along the commissures and 3–4 mm above it as well.

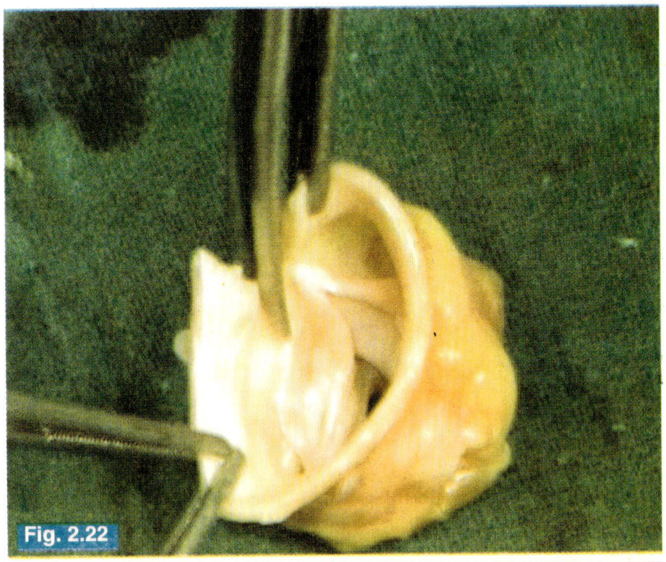

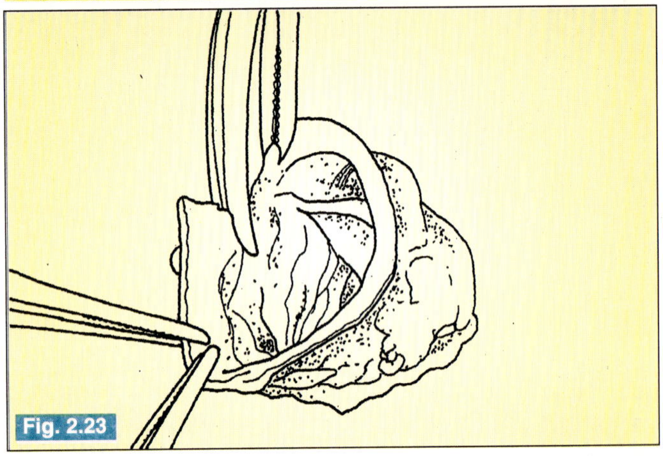

Figs 2.22, 2.23: Scalloping of the aortic homograft.

The homograft is now ready for implantation (Fig. 2.24). It may be oriented in its natural anatomic position with each sinus aligned with the appropriate sinus of the patient's aorta (homograft right coronary sinus aligned with right coronary sinus of the patient). Some surgeons prefer to rotate it about 110–120° anticlockwise aligning the left coronary sinus with the noncoronary sinus. This is said to reduce the gradient by aligning the homograft muscular bar (interventricular septum) towards the patient's anterior mitral leaflet and *vice versa*. Some surgeons also prefer to scallop only the left and right coronary sinuses and leave the noncoronary sinus intact. In that case the homograft will have to be oriented in its natural anatomic position.

Suturing

After excision of the aortic valve three 4-0 polypropylene sutures are passed through the middle of the annulus (Nadir of the sinus) of each cusp (Figs 2.25, 2.26). The needle is passed from above downwards into the left ventricle and this needle now passes into the homograft exactly below the centre of each cusp on the homograft annulus (Fig. 2.27).

In this way the cusps and commissures align with their counterparts in the patient. This may require some adjustments in bicuspid aortic valves when

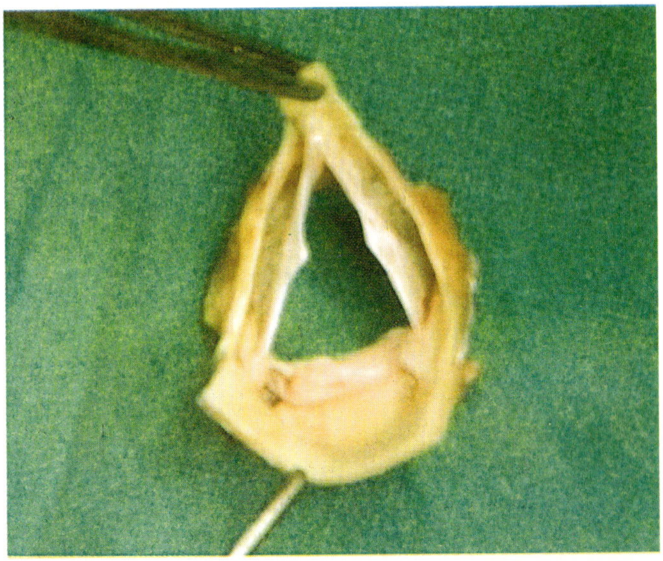

Fig. 2.24: The homograft is now ready for implantation.

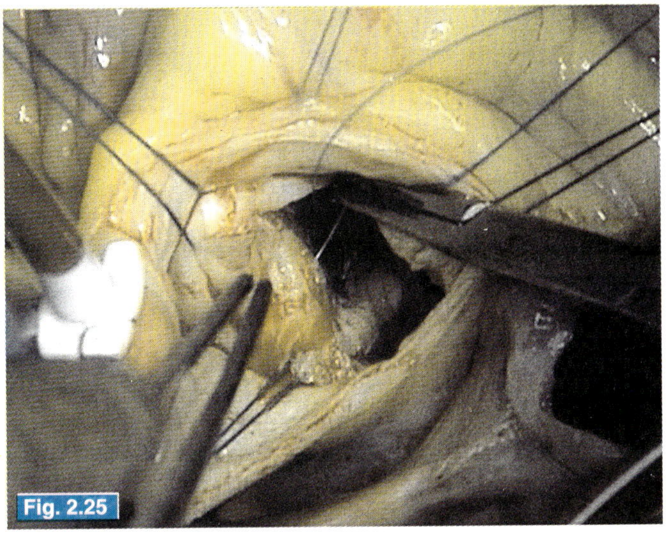

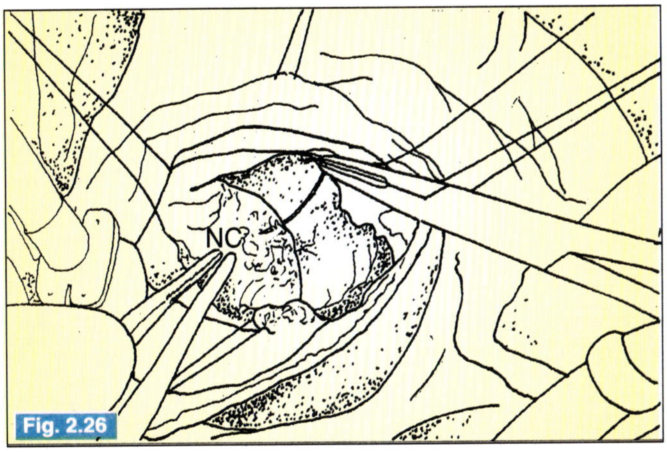

Figs 2.25, 2.26: The technique of suturing. The first 4-0 prolene suture passed through the annulus at the nadir of the left coronary sinus.

orientation of cusps and commissures requires careful assessment of the coronary ostial location.

Once all 3 sutures are taken through the homograft annulus, it is lowered into the aortic annulus. The homograft is inverted into the left ventricle. This provides a clear view of the homograft annulus for suture. Since the homograft annulus is circular, suturing requires placement of each throw carefully. Beginning on the noncoronary sinus each half of the suture now covers half of the sinus and stops short at the base of the commissure. In this way three sutures cover one-third of the circumference and are tied at the bottom of the commissures. This suture line is therefore circular. When it is completed the homograft is everted back into the aorta. This suture line can also be done by interrupted 4-0 polypropylene horizontal mattress sutures. Roughly about 12 such sutures will be required.

The top of the commissural pillars are now held taut (pulled upwards) by the assistant. A 5-0 horizontal mattress suture is taken above the top of the

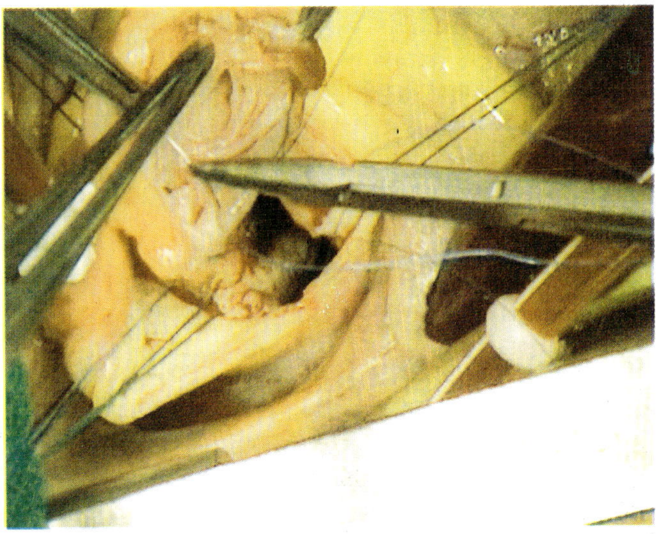

Fig. 2.27: Same suture as in Fig. 2.25 being passed through the homograft.

commissure inside out and both needles are passed through the native aorta inside out about 1 cm above the top of native valve commissure (Figs 2.28, 2.29).

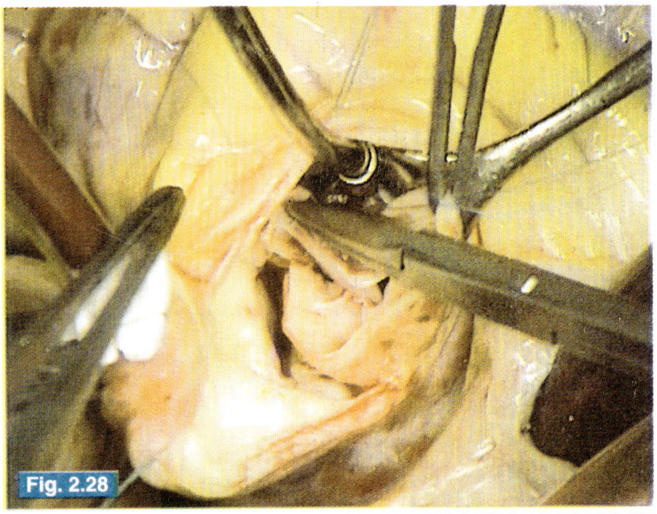

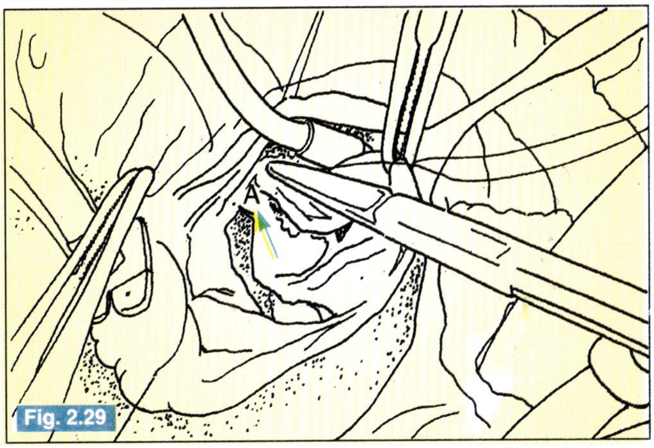

Figs 2.28, 2.29: The distal suture line. The commissural pillar (A) being pulled up.

The alignment of these commissural pillars and their anchoring at a higher level are vital details for a successful implantation. The three sutures are brought out of the aortic wall are now held on rubber shod haemostats (Figs 2.30–2.31).

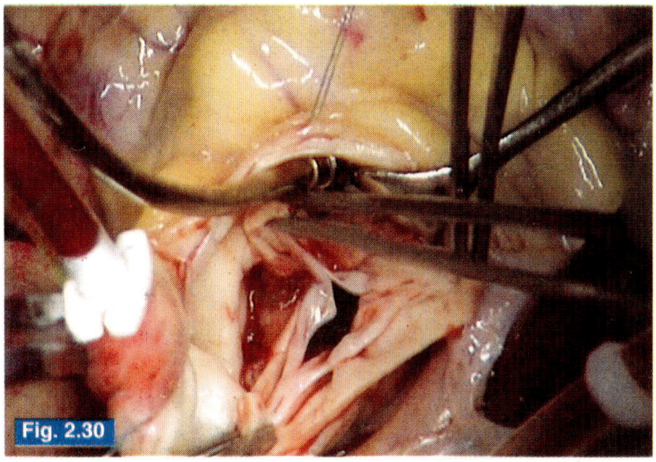

Fig. 2.30

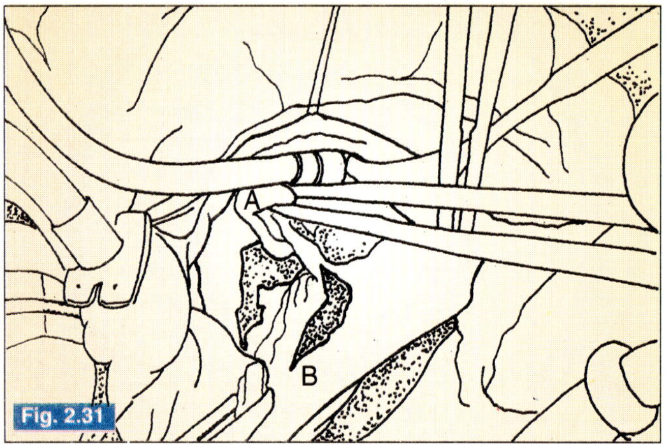

Fig. 2.31

Figs 2.30, 2.31: Fixing of all the three commissural pillars inside the aorta.

Another 5-0 polypropylene suture is taken and passed through the aortic intima 2–3 mm below the centre of the left coronary ostium (Figs 2.32, 2.33). The other needle of this suture is passed from outside in to the trimmed homograft sinus wall at the centre of the sinus. Each end is carried in a continuous fashion anchoring the scalloped homograft wall below and around the coronary ostium ascending along a curved line to the top of the commissure where it exits the aorta. The other end of the suture now ascends on the left of the left coronary ostium. Similarly another 5-0 double armed polypropylene suture anchors the scalloped right coronary sinus of the homograft to the native aortic wall below and around the right coronary ostium, one end exiting on the right and the other on the left (Figs 2.34, 2.35). The three commissural sutures are tied and

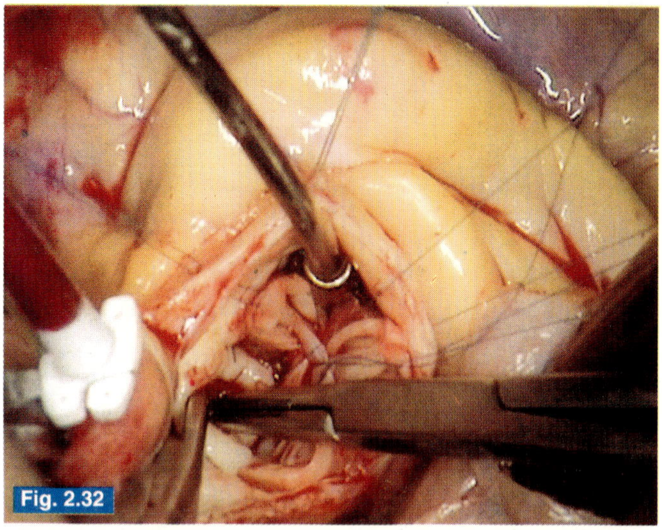

Fig. 2.32

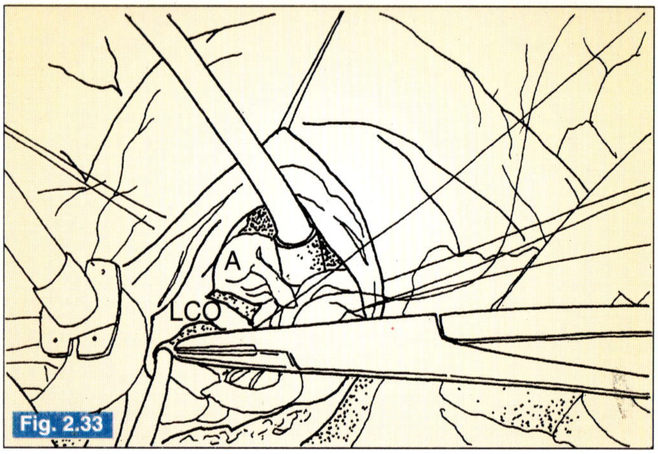

Fig. 2.33

Figs 2.32, 2.33: The beginning of the distal suture line under the left coronary ostium (LCO), note commissural pillar (A).

are tied in turn to the 5-0 continuous suture. The implantation is now complete and must be inspected to see if the coronary ostia are clearly open and that there is no damage to the cusps (Figs 2.36, 2.37).

If all 3 sinuses are scalloped a third 5-0 polypropylene completes the anchoring of the noncoronary sinus. If the noncoronary sinus is not scalloped then it is trimmed to fit the aortotomy incision. It is important to obliterate any space between the native aortic wall and the noncoronary sinus wall of the homograft. This can be accomplished while closing the aortotomy incision. Some surgeons prefer to anchor the noncoronary sinus wall with a separate suture before closing the aortotomy. The deairing protocol is as described earlier. When the heart resumes beating look for left ventricular distension due to aortic regurgitation, an indication that the valve seating is faulty. If satisfactory cardiopulmonary bypass is discontinued at 37° C. A transesophageal echocardiography is performed to assess any aortic regurgitation and to observe the new aortic valve

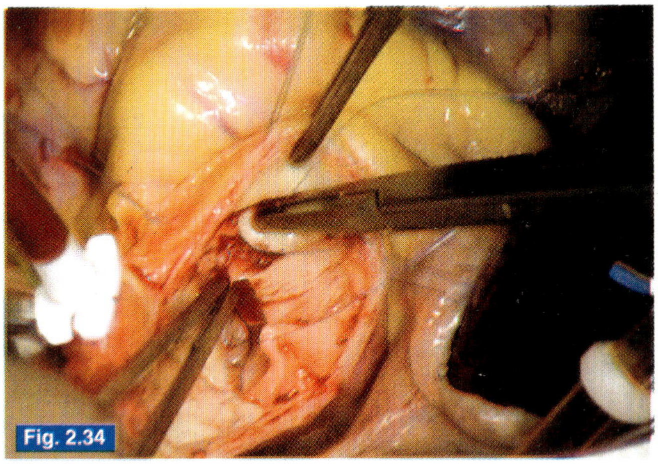

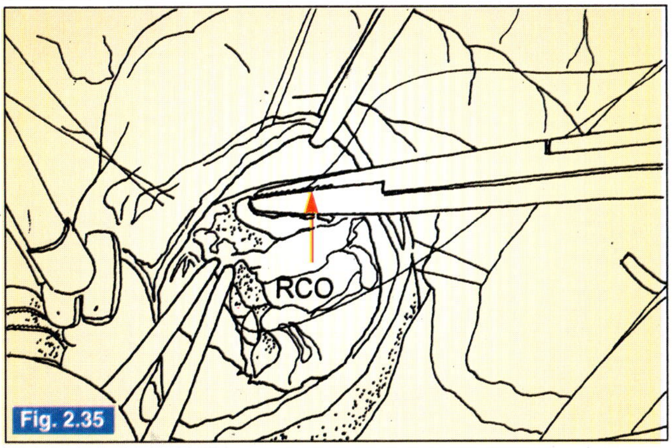

Figs 2.34, 2.35: Distal anastomosis below the right coronary ostium (RCO).

function in the short axis cross section or in the long axis section. Colour flow and Doppler echo will demonstrate any residual aortic regurgitation and any gradient across the homograft.

This technique has a learning curve because subcoronary implantation requires skill, is tricky and needs precision. If the end result is not satisfactory, it is best to resume cardiopulmonary bypass and replace the homograft with a mechanical valve.

Root Replacement Technique

This technique ensures proper geometrical alignment of the homograft without difficulty. Most surgeons therefore prefer the root replacement technique. Mark Obrien recommends that all aortic valve replacement is best performed by the root replacement technique. This does not have a learning curve like the scalloped technique. There is the possibility of calcification of the whole homograft wall when this is done in young or adolescent patients. Therefore, in India it is better to use a scallopped subcoronary technique in the young rheumatic heart disease patient so that a second operation may be safe.

As mentioned before, a transesophageal echocardiography is performed and the aortic annulus diameter is measured. There is no need to downsize the homograft if this technique is used. If a cryopreserved homograft is to be used it may be taken out for thawing. It may be the same diameter as the aortic annulus.

A midsternotomy incision is performed and the pericardium is opened in the midline. The aortic root is dissected free of the pulmonary artery. The pulmonary artery is looped carefully. Injury to the left main coronary artery is a potential hazard during this dissection.

The patient is now cannulated. A two-stage venous cannula and ascending aortic cannulae are placed. Cardiopulmonary bypass is begun. The highest point on the ascending aorta is chosen for placing the aortic vent line providing sufficient length for safe aortic clamping. Two stay sutures are placed about 4-5 mm distal to the right coronary artery origin to mark the aortotomy incision. The aorta is clamped.

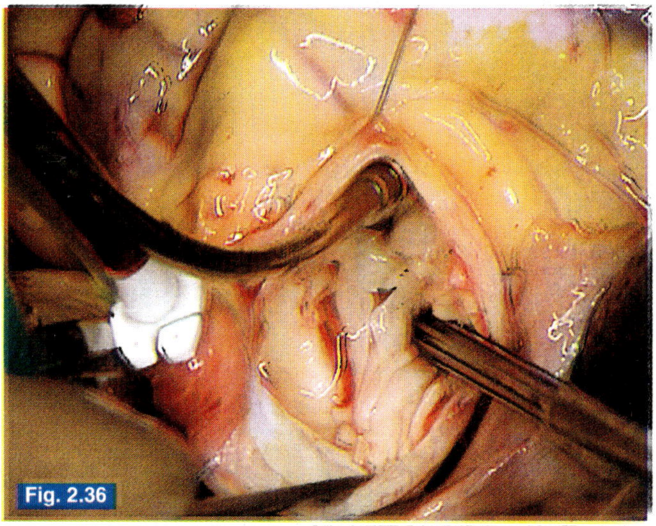

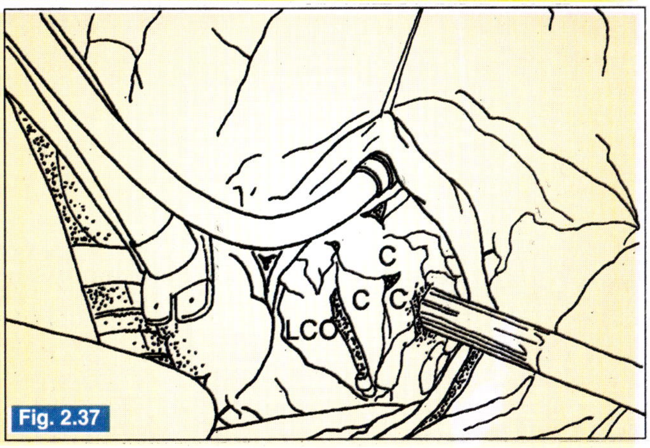

Figs 2.36, 2.37: The completed scalloped sub-coronary implantation. Note the three cusps (C) and left coronary ostium (LCO).

A vent is placed through the right superior pulmonary vein.

Aortotomy is performed between the two previously placed stay sutures. The incision is extended transversely. Care taken to avoid injury to right coronary artery ostium. Cardioplegic solution (cold blood) is injected directly into the left coronary artery and right coronary artery. Topical cooling is done with ice slush in the pericardial cavity.

Three stay sutures are placed at the commissures of the aortic valve and pulled up to the drapes. A coronary cannula is inserted in to the left coronary artery ostium to prevent debris and calcium from entering the left coronary artery. The aortic valve is excised. All calcific remnants are excised. It is not necessary to go deep into the aortic annulus or septum to remove all calcium. With this technique it can be excluded from circulation. The left ventricular cavity and ascending aorta are washed thoroughly with copious amount of cold saline — the left ventricle is squeezed gently and all the fluid is discarded through the waste suction.

The right coronary ostium is now separated as a button. The aortotomy incision is carried posteriorly. The left coronary ostium may be separated as button or left attached to the distal aorta (Elkin's technique). Ether way the left ventricle is now separated from the ascending aorta. The three aortic sinus wall remnants are excised.

The thawed aortic homograft is inspected for any damage. Excess septal muscle is trimmed carefully under vision. It is easy to damage the aortic cusps during trimming. It is, therefore, best to pass the homograft over the left thumb for this trimming.

The homograft is now oriented in its anatomic position aligning the right coronary artery and left coronary artery ostia against the patient's coronary buttons (Fig. 2.38). A slight mismatch can be corrected at anastomosis. A strip of fresh pericardium 3–4 mm in width and long enough to encircle the aortic homograft is cut out and placed around the homograft. An interrupted horizontal mattress suture technique ensures a proper anastomosis without distortion. Experienced surgeons use a continuous suture technique. For the inexperienced an interrupted suture line is recommended.

Three 4-0 polypropylene (25 mm needle) double-armed sutures are placed. The first three sutures are placed exactly at the commissures. If the native valve was bicuspid, these three sutures must be placed at equidistant points while maintaining coronary ostial alignment. These sutures are passed through and through from outside in, using the remnant of the aortic sinus to buttress the suture line. The needles are then passed inside out into the appropriate points of the homograft commissures and brought out through the pericardial strip. When all the three commissural sutures are placed the homograft is pulled away from the aortic root. Three additional sutures are placed (six needles) as horizontal mattress sutures to cover the distance between the commissural sutures. First on the right coronary sinus area, then on the left and finally on the noncoronary side. All sutures are passed outside in on the aorta and inside out under vision (especially at the belly of the homograft cusps) through the homograft and pericardial strip. The sutures are now tied. Keeping the commissural sutures on a rubber shod clamp all other suture are tied and cut. To get a completely haemostatic proximal suture line a superficial running suture on the outside from the aortic remnant through the homograft is taken and tied with the next suture.

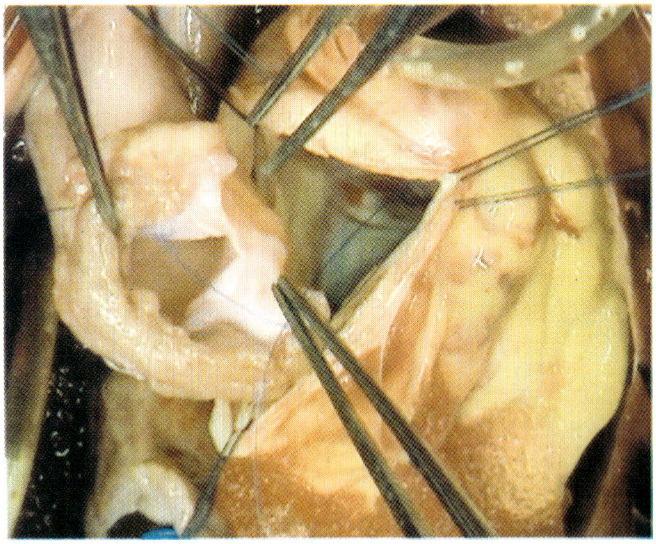

Fig. 2.38: Root replacement technique orientation of the homograft for proximal suture line.

The right coronary button is now aligned. The homograft right coronary artery site is trimmed to accommodate the patient's right coronary artery button. This suture is performed with a 4-0 (or 5-0) polypropylene (16 mm needle) in a continuous fashion beginning close to the proximal suture line. All sutures are carefully placed under vision for a proper everting anastomosis (Figs 2.39, 2.40).

The homograft is now retracted towards the heart. If the left coronary artery is trimmed as a button it is aligned with the left coronary artery ostium of the homograft which is trimmed in the correct direction to accommodate the patients' left coronary artery button without tension. Again using a 4-0 polypropylene (16 mm needle) this anastomosis is also completed with a continuous everting suture

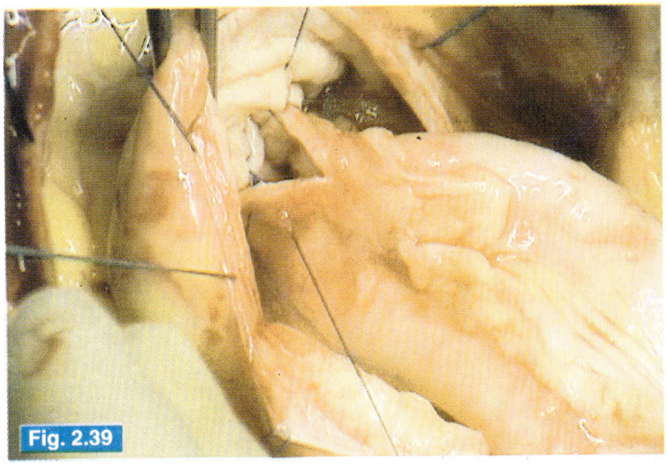

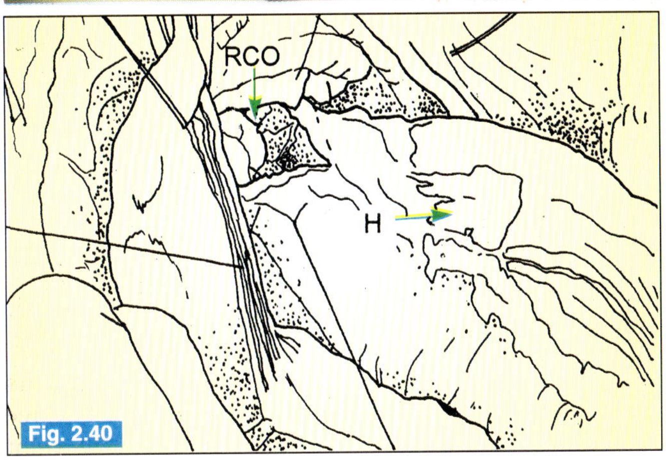

Figs 2.39, 2.40: Suture of the right coronary ostium *in situ*. Compare with Ross procedure. Right coronary ostium (RCO), homograft (H).

beginning proximally and completing distally (Figs 2.41, 2.42).

The aortic homograft is now divided at an appropriate length for the distal aorta to aorta anastomosis which commences posteriorly and ascends on either side in continuous fashion. 4-0 polypropylene (3-0 polypropylene, 25 mm needle) are used. The suture line is interrupted half way and completed anteriorly. The suture is not tied but is held on a rubber shod haemostat (Fig. 2.43).

Alternate Technique

If the left coronary artery ostium is left attached to the distal aorta then the steps change after the right coronary artery anastomosis to the homograft.

At this point the homograft is divided at an appropriate length. The posterior aortic sinus of the homograft which will receive the left coronary artery ostium is split vertically from the distal end towards the base - but stops short at least 5–6 mm distal to the attachment of the cusps. The tongue of aorta containing the left coronary artery ostium is now aligned opposite this sinus. The anastomosis begins below and ascends on either side of the split sinus in a continuous fashion. All sutures are placed from outside in (everting) under vision and close enough for a haemostatic suture line. Again this suture line

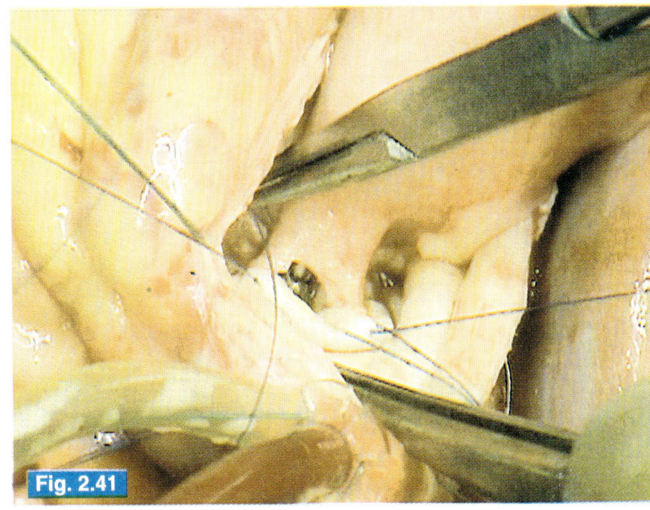

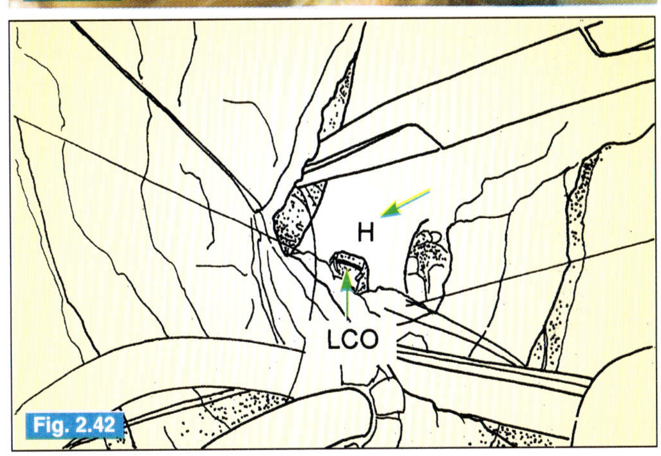

Figs 2.41, 2.42: Anastomosis of the *in situ* left coronary ostium (LCO), homograft (H).

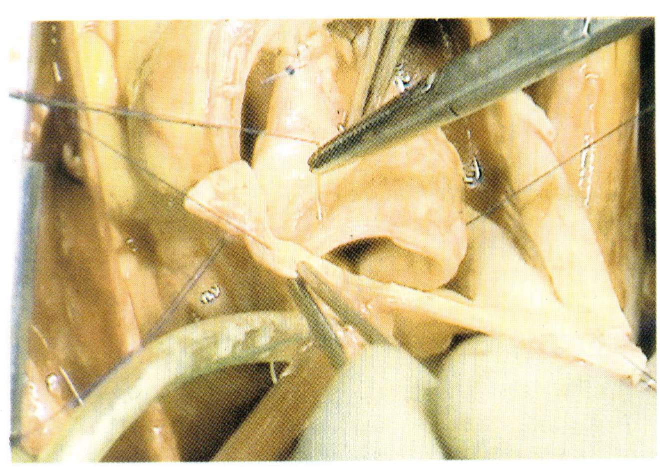

Fig. 2.43: Distal aortic homograft to aortic suture.

is also interrupted halfway and completed anteriorly as aorta–aorta anastomosis. The suture is not tied and is held on a rubber shod clamp.

The perfusionist now infuses the circulating blood into the aortic root through the aortic vent. The anterior end of the aortic suture line is left open to de air the homograft which is gently squeezed to expel all air. The suture is now pulled tight.

The homograft begins to fill and distend. All suture lines are now checked for leak. The infusion is stopped. Leaks are closed with additional sutures. when the homograft is collapsed. Now the anterior end of the suture is tied.

Deairing

The patient is rewarmed when the distal suture line is begun. The left ventricular vent is clamped. The anaesthesiologist will gently ventilate the lungs. The right hand of the surgeon is inside the pericardium squeezing the heart gently to expel all air through the aortic vent line which is open to air. The left atrial appendage is inverted. The pulmonary veins are massaged and when satisfied the head end of the patient is lowered and the aortic clamp is released slowly.

The aortic vent line is connected to cardiotomy suction and placed on strong negative suction (300 ml/min). The head end of the table is raised. The left ventricular vent is put on suction, the clamp on the venous line is released. The surgeon continues to gently massage the heart until it resumes beating or fibrillates. It is then defibrillated.

It is important to squeeze and massage the heart after releasing the aortic clamp. This will avoid distension of the left ventricle while it is rewarming and avoid left ventricular dysfunction. This is continued until the heart begins to beat or is defibrillated to sinus rhythm.

The anastomotic suture lines are now carefully checked and additional sutures are placed for haemostasis. This is done while cardiopulmonary bypass is still on so that haemostasis is secured before systemic pressure is restored. An infusion of nitroglycerine is begun at 0.025 μg/kg/min. When all is well, cardiopulmonary bypass is discontinued gradually after removing the left ventricular vent. With normal haemodynamics a transesophageal echocardiography is performed to assess homograft and left ventricular function, aortic regurgitation if any and gradient across left ventricular outflow tract. With the root replacement technique there is generally no gradient and the aortic valve is almost always competent.

Results

The operation can be performed with the same mortality as in isolated aortic valve replacement with a mechanical valve (3–5%). However, the greatest advantage is the absence of need for anticoagulation, reduced risk of thromboembolism, better haemodynamics combined with the disadvantage of limited durability. One distinct advantage is the retention of life span, a low postoperative attrition rate compared to aortic valve replacement with a mechanical valve.

Aortic Valve Repair

This operation is indicated in patients with normal or near normal aortic valve morphology such as in patients with congenital heart disease like ventricular septal defect + aortic regurgitation. It is also indicated in patients with ruptured belly of aortic valve cusps in bacterial endocarditis. It can also be performed in a select group of patients with rheumatic heart disease. Several techniques have been described by Carpentier, Duran, Cosgrove, Trusler and others. However, the ultimate decision to repair rests with the surgeon of the day.

Assessment of reparability is best done with echocardiography (transthoracic and trans-esophageal echocardiography). A prolapsing cusp in ventricular septal defect/aortic regurgitation, a perforated cusp in subacute bacterial endocarditis, thickened and rolled out cusps in rheumatic heart disease can be visualised. Aortic regurgitation can be quantified. Visual assessment at surgery provides the best opportunity for repair. It is best to acquire the ability to perform transesophageal echocardiography which will enhance the surgeon's ability to assess reparability.

Techniques

A midsternotomy incision is made. The pericardium is opened in the midline and tacked up to the drapes with stay sutures. The external appearance of the heart is assessed. There is left ventricular enlargement, a large bouncy aortic root and an enlarged pulmonary artery in patients with ventricular septal defect and/or pulmonary hypertension. A systolic thrill may be present over the aorta indicating a large forward flow. A systolic thrill over the right ventricular outflow tract may be due to a ventricular septal defect.

Cardiopulmonary bypass is established with aortic and right atrial cannulation with two stage (superior vena cava and inferior vena cava are cannulated separately if there is a ventricular septal defect), the aortic vent line is placed high on the aorta. Aortotomy site (1 cm distal to right coronary artery) is marked by stay suture. A left atrial vent is placed through right superior pulmonary vein. Normothermic perfusion is combined with direct antegrade cardioplegia delivery and topical ice slush for myocardial protection. Retrograde cardioplegia through the coronary sinus can also be used with the disadvantage that the coronary return to the aorta would be annoying at times. Cardioplegia infusion is repeated every 20 minutes (maximum interval at normothermic perfusion).

The aortic valve is delivered into the aortotomy incision with traction on the commissural sutures. The valve cusps are inspected. A ventricular septal defect, if present, is located and assessed for size and morphology. A patch is usually recommended for closing such a ventricular septal defect. The subvalvular aortic outlet is examined for endocardial thickening and septal hypertrophy. During ventricular septal defect closure the aortic cusps are best retracted with a 6-0 polypropylene stay suture placed at the central lunule and weighed down with a rubber shod light weight artery forceps.

After completion of ventricular septal defect closure the commissural stay sutures are released dropping the aortic valve into its normal anatomic position. A 6-0 polypropylene suture (double-armed) is taken and the needles passed through the central lunule of each cusps thus closing the aortic valve. With gentle traction on this suture (Frater's stitch) the free edge of each cusp can be seen and any redundancy between the central suture and the commissure is noted and the length of redundancy is assessed by holding the free edge at the commissure and folding it. This manoeuvre will demonstrate both the cusp and the site where a repair will be required. The redundancy may affect one or more regions.

A commissural placation is now performed as described by Trusler. A 5-0 polypropylene double-arm suture buttressed with a piece of pericardium is passed through the redundant free edge and brought out through the aortic wall. This folds the free edge and the second needle passes through the fold and is also brought out of the aorta and tied on a piece of Teflon felt. This commissural plication is covered by a hood created by a piece of pericardium folded over it and fixed with a 5-0 polypropylene vertical mattress suture. The central (Frater's) stitch is placed on traction and any further redundancy can be repaired in similar fashion. Finally the Frater's stitch is removed.

Cusp Resection

When a large redundancy and prolapse of the cusp into the left ventricular outflow tract is noted, it may be partially resected. A wedge-shaped central portion of the cusp from the free edge to about the middle of the cusp is excised and the defect is repaired with 6-0 (5-0) vertical mattress sutures.

Subcommissural Annuloplasty

Coaptation of the cusps can be improved by reducing the diameter of the sinotubular junction (Duran). A 5-0 polypropylene pledgeted suture is taken 4-5 mm away on the sinus wall, at the level of the commissure. This suture is passed from outside in a vertical mattress fashion (Fig. 2.44). The needles are then passed through the aortic intima underneath the commissural pillar. It is then passed 5–6 mm away from the commissure at the same level and passed through the aortic wall from inside out and tied on a pledget outside the aorta. This will reduce the sinotubular diameter by 1 cm and pushes the commissures forward. This can be performed if necessary at all the three commissures. Care must be taken to ensure that there is no damage to the cusps or the coronary ostia.

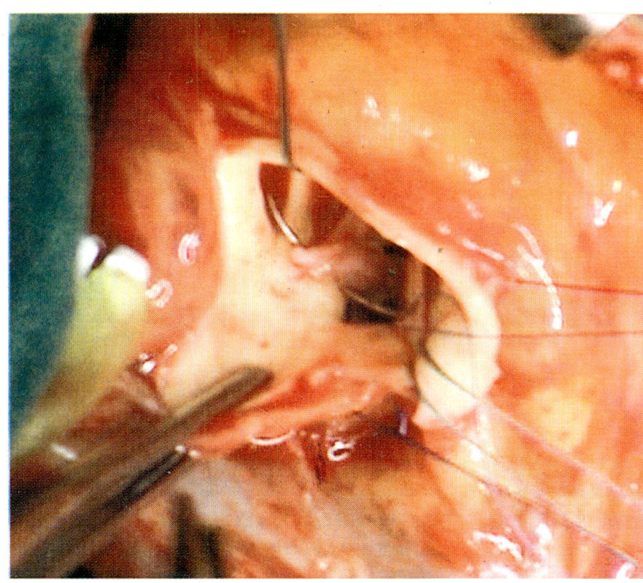

Fig. 2.44: The technique of sub-commissural annuloplasty.

Cusp Refixation

Occasionally a bicuspid aortic cusp (thin and pliable) may detach from the aortic wall (at the rudimentary third commissures). Occasionally a central chord-like raphe supporting the bicuspid cusp from prolapsing may rupture. In both of these conditions the aortic valve competence can be restored by refixing the cusps at the appropriate site with pericardium buttressed 5-0 polypropylene sutures.

Circumferential Annuloplasty

In patients with a dilated aortic annulus competence can be restored by an encircling annuloplasty suture (Carpentier). This suture begins from the base of the noncoronary cusp. The two needles are passed from outside in, into the left ventricular outflow tract. One needle now runs gathering the aortic annulus in a purse-string fashion with the needle passing below the attachment of the cusp at the base of the commissural triangle and brought out of the aorta at the commissure between the right and left cusps between the aorta and pulmonary artery. The left half of the suture runs in a similar fashion below the left half of the noncoronary cusp and below the left coronary cusp and exits at the same point outside the aorta. This suture buttressed with a pledget at both ends is tightened over a large size Hegar dilator (19–25) passed into the left ventricular outflow tract and tied while the dilator remains in the left ventricular outflow tract. The dilator is now removed.

Cusp Thinning (Cusp unrolling)

This procedure dramatically restores the normal architecture of the aortic cusps and is useful especially in the thickened fused cusps of rheumatic aortic regurgitation.

Using the tip of a sharp No. 11 blade the cusps are separated at the commissure by careful incision (Fig. 2.45). A right-angled forceps is inserted through valve into the left ventricular outflow tract to grasp the thickened endocardium below the commissure and the belly of the cusp. Gentle traction usually separates if from the normal left ventricular endocardium. The right angle clamp is now withdrawn. The surgeon holds the separated endocardium below the valve commissure with a tissue forceps and using upward traction gently coaxes this material to separate from the underlying normal cusp assisting with another tissue forceps in the other hand.

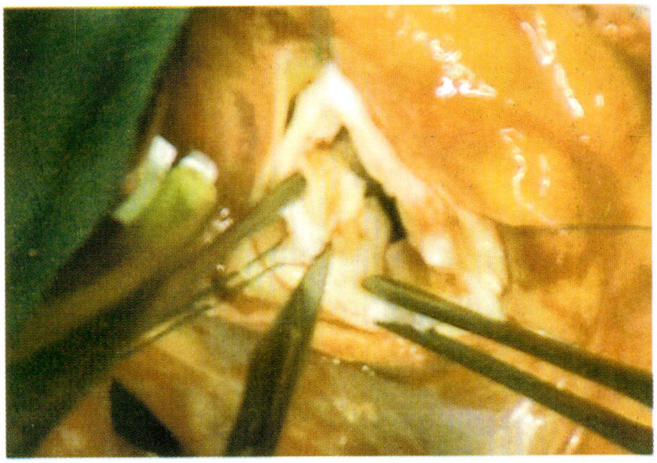

Fig. 2.45: Aortic commissural incision. Note the thickened cusps.

Patient, gentle, traction dissection removes this fibrocalcific peel from the cusps almost like a cast. This is excised at the top of the free edge of each cusp, leaving the underlying cusps looking almost normal, thin and pliable. If a central aortic regurgitation is suspect, one of the two annuloplasty (subcommissure or circumferential) procedures may restore competence of the aortic valve.

Cusp Extension

With gluteraldehyde tanned autologous pericardium cusp extension may be performed if the cusps are contracted and retracted (rheumatic heart disease). Using a frater's stitch the radius of the aorta is measured at the free edge level. Double this figure will be the length of the pericardial patch. The shape is an ellipse (or quarter moon) and the width is measured at the centre of the cusp to bring it up to the other cusp free edge.

A rectangular piece of pericardium is cleaned of all fibrofatty tissue and immersed in 0.625% buffered gluteraldehyde solution for 10 min. An elliptical piece is cut out from this as measured. It is then sutured to the remaining free edge of the cusp using a 5-0 polypropylene suture in a continuous fashion. The suture is brought out of the aorta at the commissure and the commissural end is reinforced with another 5-0 polypropylene suture.

In most patients a combination of all the above techniques can generally restore competence. Also a perfectly competent valve following these reparative procedures is nearly impossible to obtain. Trivial to mild aortic regurgitation should be considered as a good result if there is no gradient (rarely found).

Aortic valve repair is a difficult operation. It requires **imagination, skill, courage** and the **conviction** to accept less than a perfect result. However, it has the potential to restore normal function without gradient permitting growth of the aortic valve and annulus while avoiding anticoagulation. Most surgeons lack the confidence to attempt. A repair does not pose a problem if it fails. The valve can still be replaced without increasing mortality or morbidity.

Postoperative assessment must be performed before heparin reversal. The most reliable method is transesophageal echocardiography. Observing left atrial vent return, distension of left ventricle, aortic diastolic pressure, etc. are unreliable for assessment of residual aortic regurgitation. When a satisfactory result is noted on transesophageal echocardiography, the patient can be decannulated and heparin reversed. Again closing the pericardium is indeed required in these patients for a safe reoperation.

Results

Repair of aortic valve provides a satisfactory result. Most surgeons agree and demonstrate good long-term (10–20 yr) reoperation-free, symptom-free survival in patients with ventricular septal defect aortic regurgitation. However, durability of repair is not yet conclusively demonstrated in other aetiologies especially in rheumatic heart disease. Repairability may be about 70% in rheumatic heart disease. Of those who have good result at surgery, 10% will require reoperation within 10 years. The reasons for reoperation are many including technical failure, degeneration, recurrence of rheumatic heart disease, etc.

In India, aortic valve repair should occupy a prominent place in the surgeons' desirable skills because of the young age of these patients with rheumatic heart disease. A 5–10 year event-free/ reoperation-free result in 70% of patients will still permit the advantages enumerated for these patients, especially when homograft valve banks are scarce.

Aortic Valve Replacement with Pulmonary Autograft (Ross Procedure)

This operation is ideally suited for patients with congenital aortic valve stenosis, bicuspid aortic valve with aortic stenosis and for rheumatic aortic regurgitation (with or without aortic stenosis) in older patients. It is recommended if the aortic annulus diameter is less than 30 mm and if the pulmonary valve is about the same size and has normal tricuspid morphology and function. It is not suitable for young rheumatic heart disease patients (less than 35 years) especially if additional mitral valve pathology exists.

Preoperative Transesophageal Echocardiography

The aortic valve is visualised in the short axis and in the long-axis 4 chamber views. The aortic annulus is sized. The pulmonary valve is visualised in the short axis view, annulus size and cusp morphology are assessed.

A midsternotomy incision is made. The pericardium is opened towards the right, leaving a large flap attached to the left half. External cardiac anatomy is assessed. The ascending aorta and pulmonary artery are carefully separated by sharp dissection. The aorta is looped and retracted to the right. The main pulmonary artery, bifurcation and right pulmonary artery are mobilised. The main pulmonary artery is carefully looped avoiding any injury to the left main coronary artery posteriorly. It is then lifted and separated from the back of the right ventricular outflow tract, carefully till the right ventricular outflow tract muscle is visible. A marker stitch is placed on the main pulmonary artery 2–3 mm distal to the sinuses.

Cardiopulmonary bypass is established with ascending aortic and bicaval cannulae. It is not necessary to loop the superior vena cava and inferior vena cava. An aortic vent is placed at its highest point on the ascending aorta. Aortotomy site is marked by two stay sutures 4–5 mm distal to the right coronary artery origin. Cardiopulmonary bypass is begun and patient is cooled to 32°C. A vent is placed in the right superior pulmonary vein. Aorta is crossclamped and aortotomy incision is made and extended in to the noncoronary sinus. Cardioplegia is delivered directly into the coronary ostia, ice slush is used for topical cooling.

Three stay sutures are placed on the aortic commissures and pulled up to the drapes. The aortic valve is excised and the calcium is carefully removed with care to protect the left main coronary artery ostium. The left ventricle and ascending aorta are washed thoroughly with copious amounts of fluid. The aortic annulus is sized with conical graduated sizer.

Autograft Harvesting

(See under mitral valve replacement with autograft.)

Autograft Implantation

The autograft may be implanted with three different techniques. A scalloped subcoronary implantation (described earlier in homograft aortic valve replacement) or a mini root (intra-aortic) or as a full root.

The scallopped subcoronary technique is a bit difficult and has a learning curve. The mini root technique is not popular for the autograft implantation. The complete root replacement technique has been the most universally used method.

Root Replacement Technique

After excision of the aortic valve when autograt harvesting is done attention is now focused on aortic root. The right coronary artery ostium is separated as a button (Fig. 2.46). The left coronary artery ostium is retained with the distal aorta as a tongue (Fig. 2.47). The noncoronary sinus is trimmed. The double armed 4-0 polypropylene sutures are taken from outside into the aortic annulus using the aortic sinus remnant to reinforce. The three sutures are placed at equidistant points so that the right coronary artery ostium and left coronary artery ostium will be positioned in the centre of the corresponding sinus. If the native aortic valve (excised) was tricuspid then the natural commissures are used.

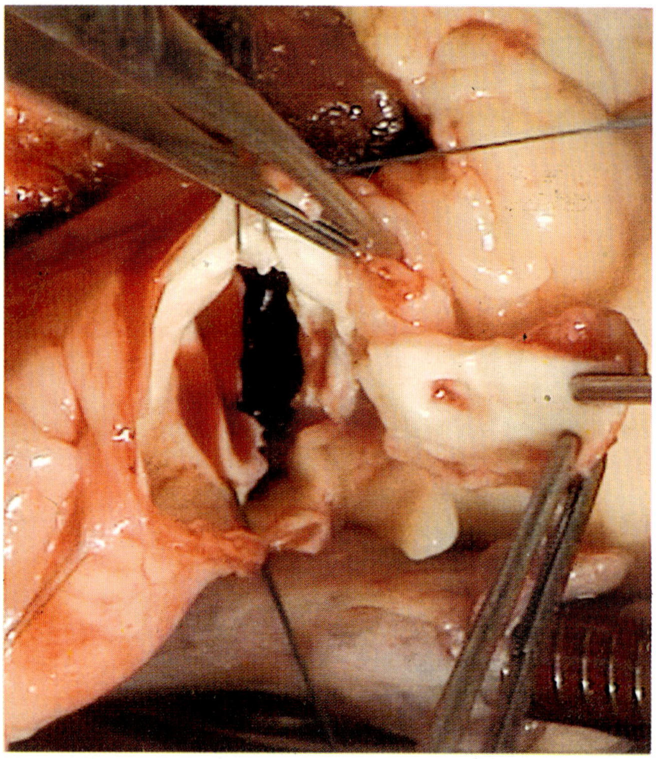

Fig. 2.46: Separated right coronary ostium as a button.

Three additional sutures are passed from inside the aortic annulus at the right coronary sinus and brought out of the aorta. These double-armed needle are now passed through the septum and into the right ventricular outflow tract 2–3 mm proximal to the divided end and retained on haemostats. These are for later anastomosis of the pulmonary homograft and they provide an excellent haemostatic suture line (Fig. 2.48).

The three aortic commissural sutures are now passed through the autograft exactly below the commisssures retaining the anterior and posterior

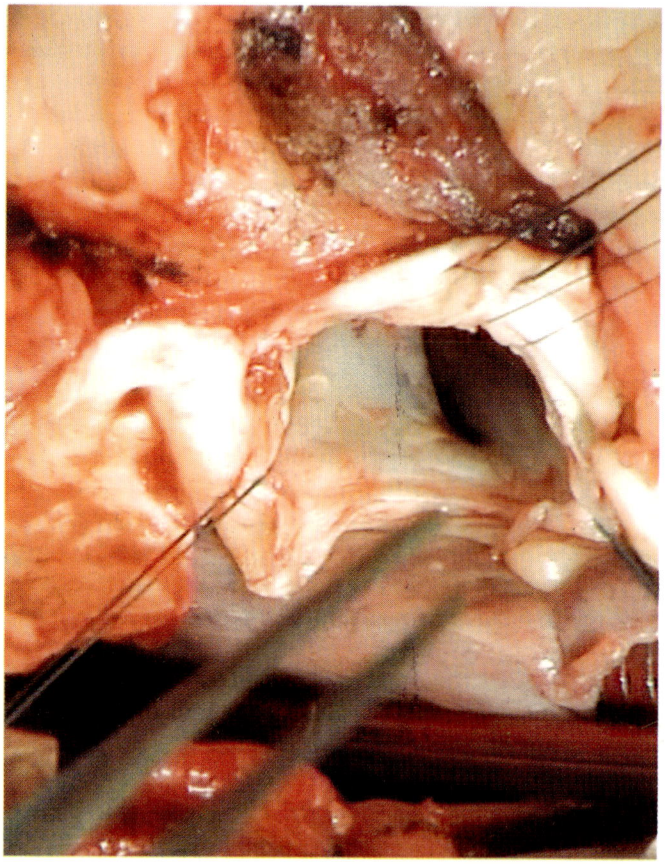

Fig. 2.47: Left coronary ostium retained with the distal aorta.

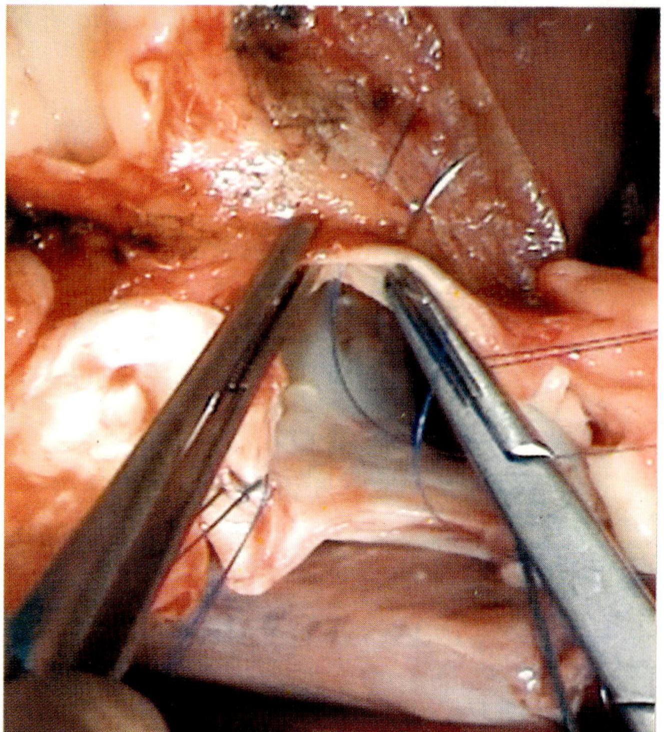

Fig. 2.48: Horizontal mattress sutures of polypropylene passed from inside the aorta across the septum to the right ventricle. These are for the homograft anastomosis.

aspects of the pulmonary artery in the same orientation. A 3–4 mm wide fresh pericardial strip is used to buttress this suture line by passing the double needles through the pericardial strip. When all three sutures are placed correctly through the autograft, the autograft is lowered to the aortic annulus.

This proximal autograft anastomosis must be in the exact anatomical position as the native aortic valve annulus. If the right ventricular outflow tract muscle is sutured instead, there is a greater likelihood of autograft dilatation postoperatively.

The autograft is now inverted into the left ventricular outflow tract. The suture between the left and the right sinus is now tied over the pericardial strip. It is then run in a continuous fashion in an anticlockwise direction to complete the posterior (left coronary sinus) suture (Figs 2.49, 2.50). All throws of the suture are placed under direct vision avoiding injury to the autograft cusps. The loops are now lightened using a nerve hook. The second suture at the commissure between left coronary and non-coronary sinuses is now tied and one short end of this is tied to the first suture and held on a haemostat.

The other end of the first suture now proceeds in a clockwise direction in the right coronary sinus area again as a continuous loop, placed under vision. The loops are tightened with a nerve hook and the suture is held by an assistant. The third suture at the commissure between the right coronary and noncoronary sinuses is now tied and the short end is tied with the end of the first suture. Using the two long ends of the second and third sutures in the noncoronary sinus area, the proximal suture line is completed about the middle of the noncoronary sinus. The loops are tightened and the suture is tied down. It is important to reinforce this suture line on the native side with the remnant of the aortic wall and on the autograft side with a piece of pericardium in adults.

In infants and children interrupted double armed mattress sutures are used and no pericardial strip is used. This is to permit growth and avoid stenosis.

The autograft is now everted. It is preferable to complete the distal autograft to aorta anastomosis and autograft to left coronary artery anastomosis before the right coronary artery ostium is anastomosed.

The posterior sinus of the autograft is now split vertically to receive the tongue of distal aorta with the left coronary artery ostium (Figs 2.51, 2.52). The suture begins below the left coronary artery ostium. The needles are passed from 'outside in' in posterior sinus the autograft and from 'inside out'

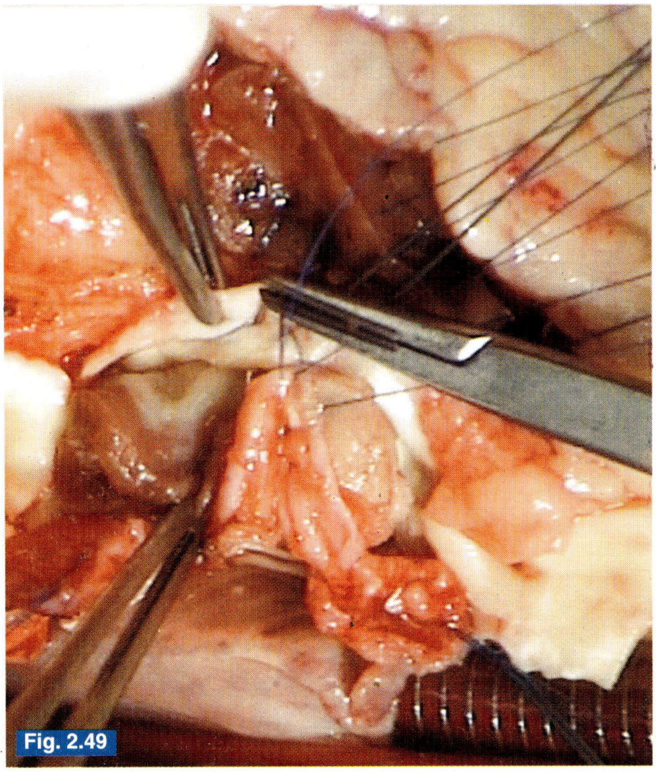

Fig. 2.49

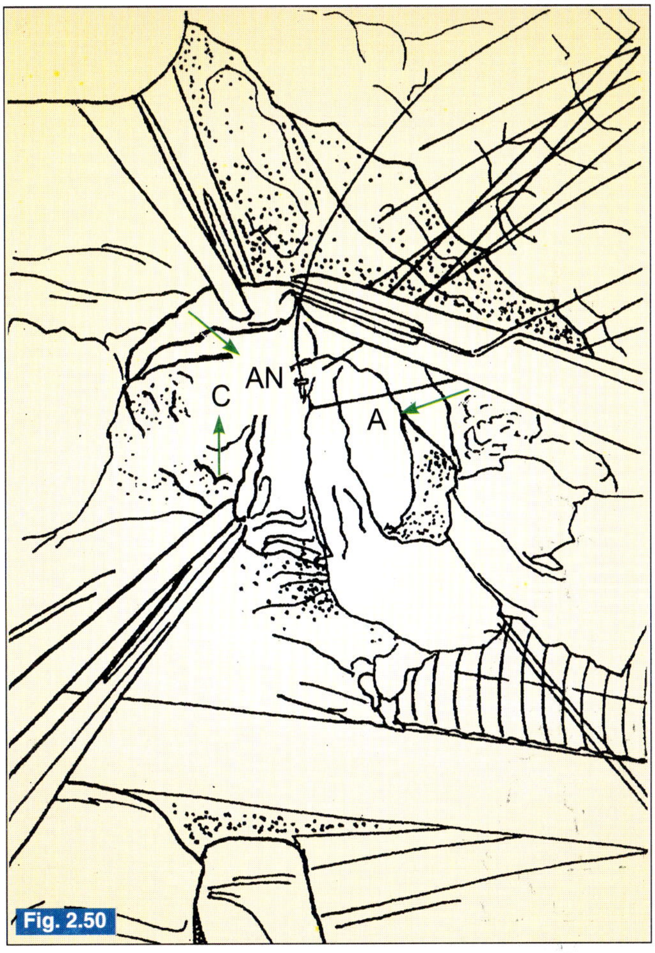

Fig. 2.50

Figs 2.49, 2.50: The inverted autograft (A) being sutured to remnant of aortic annulus (AN). Note the autograft cusp (C).

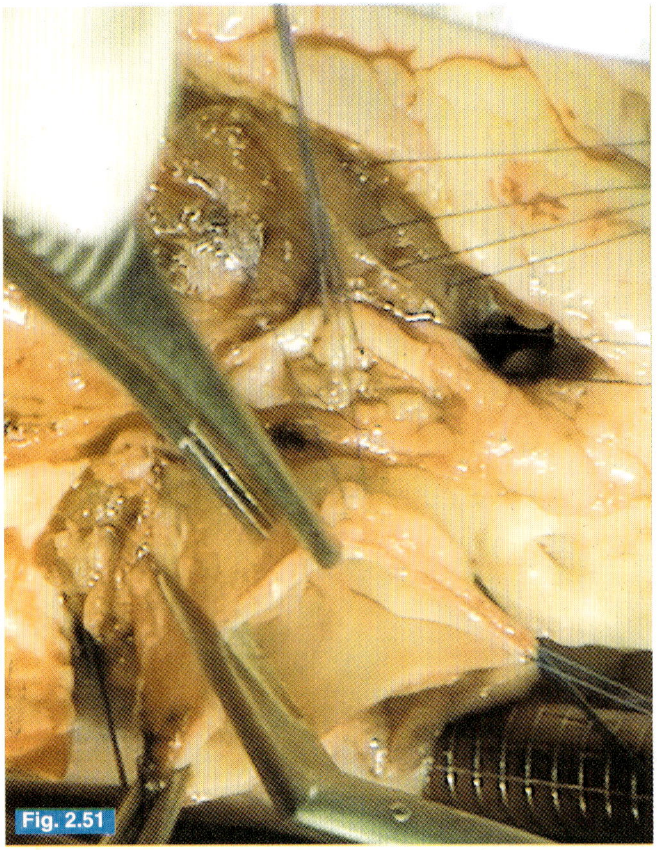

Fig. 2.51

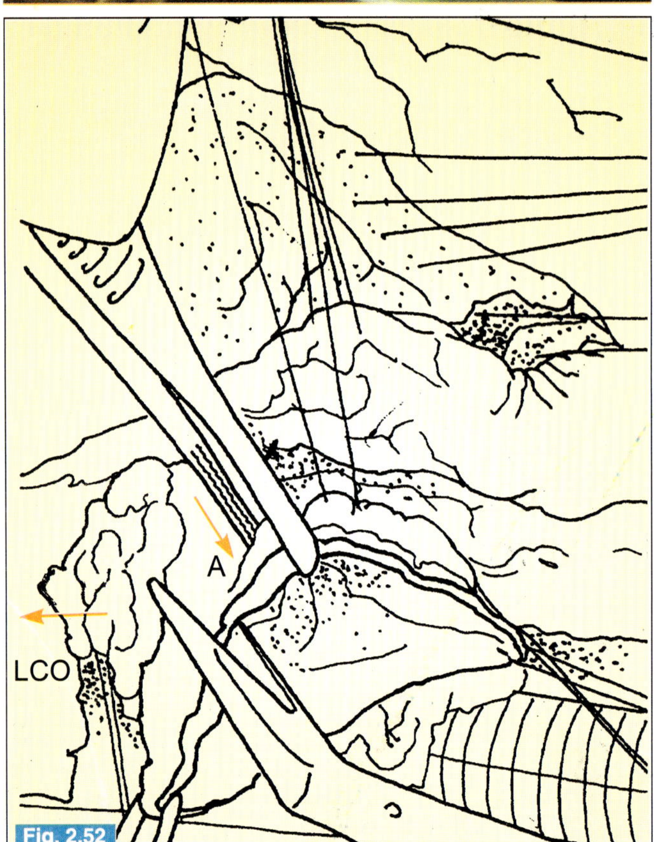

Fig. 2.52

Figs 2.51, 2.52: Splitting of the posterior sinus wall of the autograft (A) to accommodate the left coronary ostium (LCO) for the distal anastomosis.

in the distal aorta. The two ends are now used to carefully anastomose the autograft with the aorta placing all sutures in an everting haemostatic suture line (Fig. 2.53). This is interrupted midway on both the right and left side and tied to an additional 4-0 polypropylene suture. The long end of the new suture from either side completes the autograft to aorta distal anastomosis anteriorly (Figs 2.54, 2.55). The suture is not tied. The cardioplegia line is connected to the aortic vent and the perfusionist is asked to fill the ascending aorta. Air is evacuated from the loose anterior suture line. When the autograft is deaired, this suture is tightened. The autograft now begins to distend. The sinuses bulge. The location of the right coronary ostium is now determined and while the autograft is distended an incision is made at the selected spot on the right coronary sinus of the autograft. Using a punch this opening is enlarged. All blood is sucked out and infusion is stopped. The right coronary artery button is now carefully anastomosed to the autograft under vision by a continuous 5-0 suture (Fig. 2.56). It is important to trim the right coronary artery button and not to make it too large. This way injury to the autograft cusps is avoided at this step. The autograft anastomosis is now complete and further cardioplegic infusion is made into the neo aortic

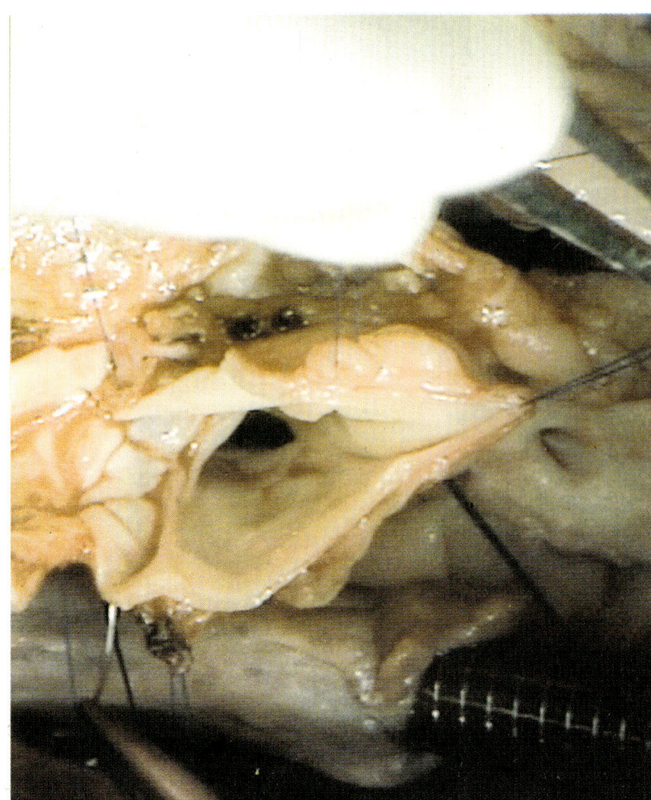

Fig. 2.53: The posterior sinus anastomosis.

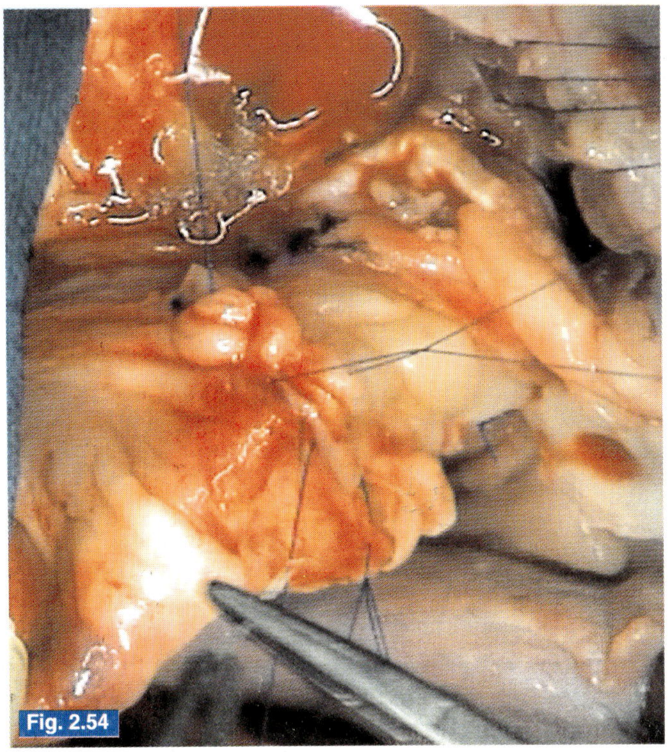

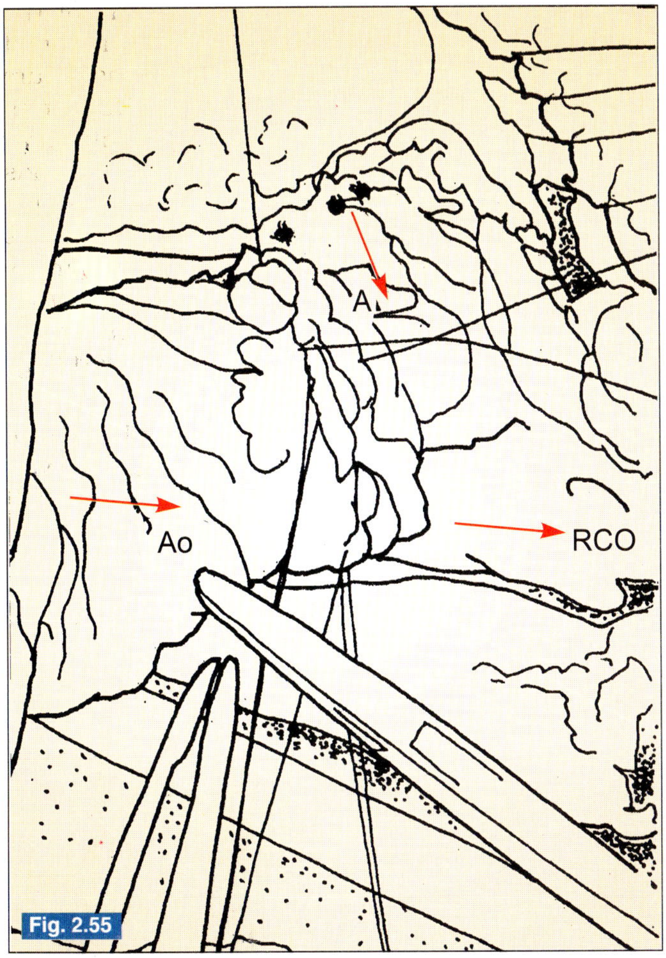

Figs 2.54, 2.55: Completed distal anastomosis between autograft (A) and aorta (Ao). Note the right coronary button (RCO).

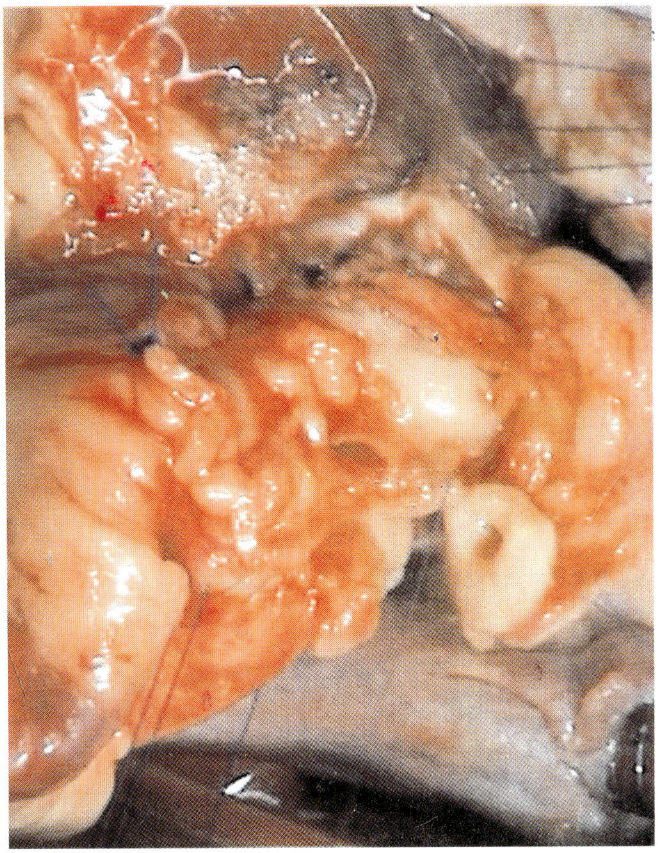

Fig. 2.56: Anastomosis of right coronary ostium to the autograft.

root. This will also provide an opportunity to inspect the suture line for haemostasis.

Right Ventricular Outflow Tract Reconstruction

The raw posterior surface of the right ventricular outflow tract is sometimes a source of troublesome bleeding. This area is difficult to visualise after completion of the procedure. In addition any sutures placed blindly to control bleeding can easily cause injury to the left main coronary artery, left anterior descending or the first septal artery. A technique to avoid bleeding complications had been described previously.

An elliptical piece of the remnant of the aortic sinus wall or a piece of pericardium is sutured to this raw surface so that it is covered (Figs 2.57, 2.58). A 5-0 polypropylene suture begins at the far left side and proceeds to take the epicardial fat. The needle bites are taken under vision to avoid injury to the left main coronary artery, left anterior descending and septal branches. The pericardial patch is placed with its smooth side upwards. The suture line comes forwards to include the intimal surface of the cut edge of the right ventricular outflow tract. Before

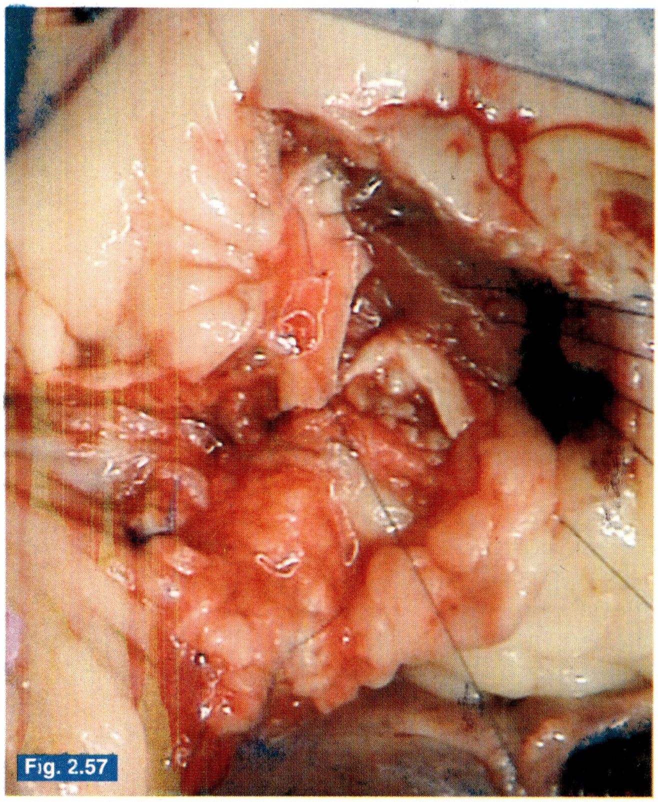

Fig. 2.57

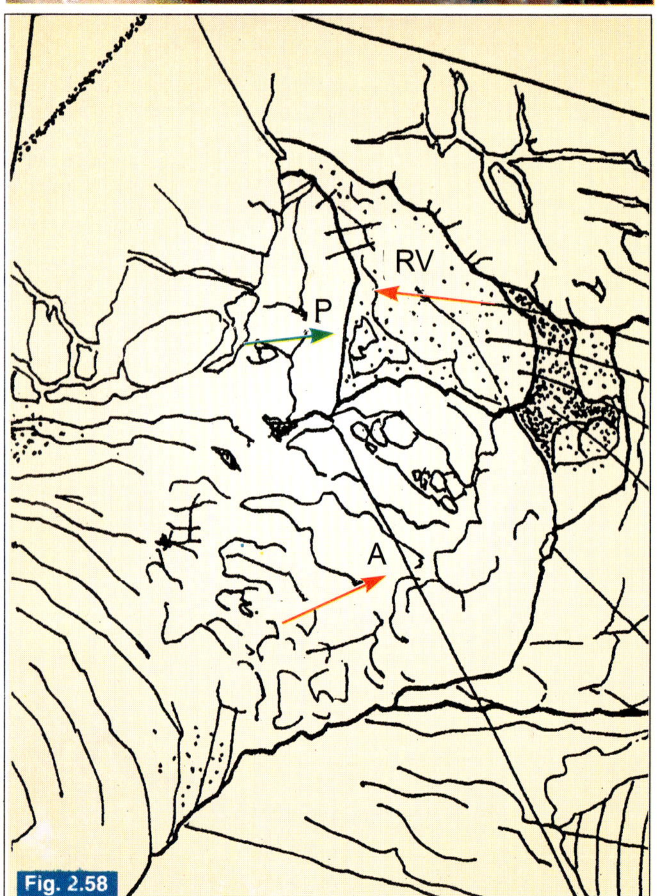

Fig. 2.58

Figs 2.57, 2.58: Covering of the raw posterior surface of the right ventricular outflow tract with a pericardial patch (P); right ventricle (RV), autograft (A).

tying this suture a piece of thymus is placed under the patch for haemostasis. The suture is then tied.

Pulmonary Homograft Anastomosis

Two 4-0 polypropylene sutures are passed from the pericardial patch on right ventricular outflow tract into the right ventricle as a horizontal mattress suture. The sutures are placed to the left of the 3 other sutures placed previously and held on haemostats. The pulmonary homograft is now placed on the right ventricular surface in a inverted position with its posterior surface facing upwards and the distal pulmonary artery end towards the apex of the heart. A 4–5 mm wide strip of pericardium is taken and an assistant grips the homograft and pericardium together.

The horizontal mattress sutures are now passed through the homograft proximal end and through the strip of pericardium. When all sutures have been placed the homograft is lowered and the sutures are tied. The first and last sutures are now carried forwards anteriorly. The homograft is now flipped up towards the pulmonary artery aligning the anterior cut end of the right ventricular outflow tract with the anterior wall of the homograft. This suture line can be completed in a continuous fashion from the right and left corners. The right ventricular outflow tract is inspected and any muscle bands likely to produce obstruction are divided under vision before the anastomosis is begun. The suture line is completed anteriorly. This way the pulmonary homograft is aligned in its anatomical position and on completion of the anastomosis appears similar to the natural external appearance of the heart (Figs 2.59, 2.60).

The venous line is partially clamped and the pulmonary homograft distal end is held closed with the vascular forceps. When this distends the length required is determined and the homograft pulmonary artery is divided at an appropriate length. The clamp on the venous line is removed. The distal pulmonary to pulmonary anastomosis is now begun. A 4-0 polypropylene suture is passed through the homograft pulmonary artery outside in and taken inside out of the native pulmonary artery. Both needles are passed in this way. The right needle is now used to begin this anastomosis on the aortic side and ascends gathering the adventitia of the patients pulmonary artery. This suture line is interrupted half way at about 10 O'clock position. The left needle is now used to complete the lateral quarter of the posterior wall anastomosis and this is interrupted at about 2 O'clock position. The anterior suture line is now completed coming forwards from the right and left towards the centre of the

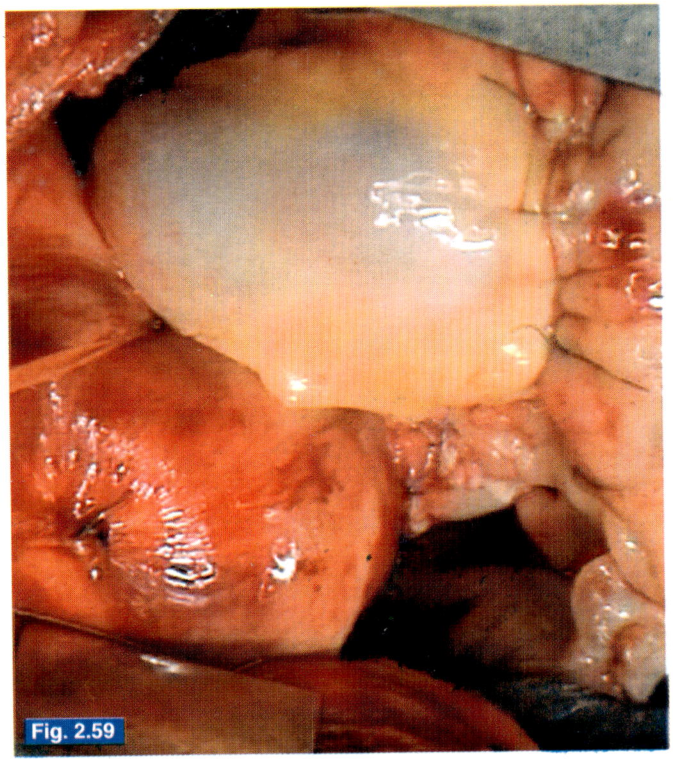

Fig. 2.59

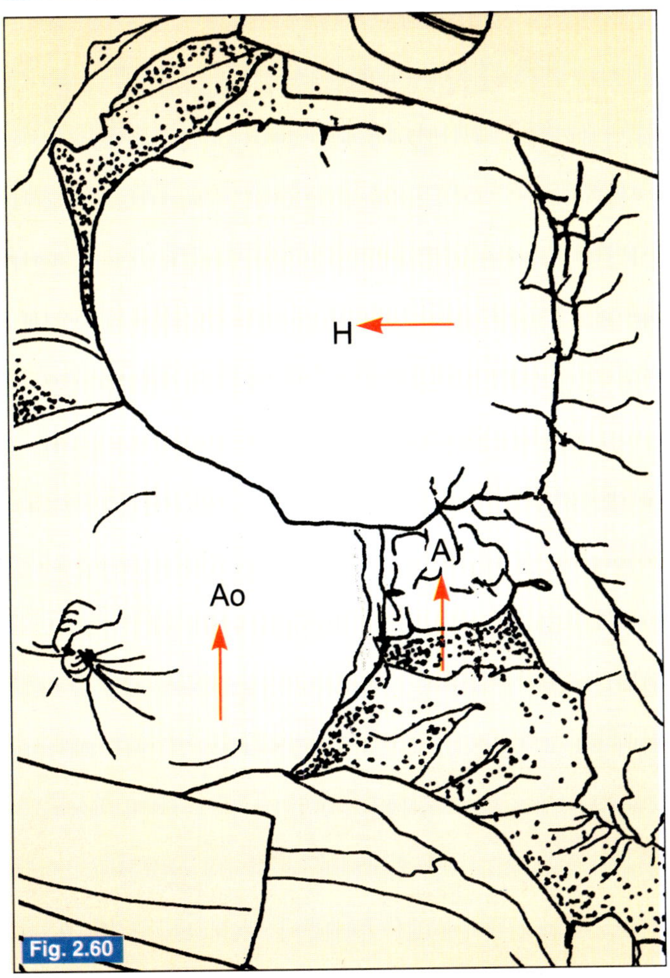

Fig. 2.60

Figs 2.59, 2.60: Completed Ross procedure. Note aorta (Ao), pulmonary homograft (H) and autograft (A).

patients pulmonary artery. The heart is filled and the right ventricle and right atrium are deaired before tying this suture.

During the right ventricular outflow tract reconstruction the patient is rewarmed. The aortic vent line is connected to cardiotomy sucker through a three-way stopcock. When the patient is rewarmed to 37°C the left atrial vent is clamped.

Deairing

The surgeon's right hand is inserted into the pericardial cavity. The inferior vena cava cannula is clamped. The anaesthetist begins gentle ventilation of the lungs. The hand gently messages the left ventricle, the right and left pulmonary veins and the left atrium posteriorly. Air is evacuated through the aortic vent line until a continuous stream of blood flows out of the three-way stopcock. When all air is evacuated the aortic clamp is released. The aortic vent is placed on negative suction (300 ml/min). The surgeon continues to gently massage the heart and remove the clamp on the venous line and the left atrial vent is placed on negative suction.

When cardiac action begins spontaneously or after defibrillation the aortic vent suction is increased to 300 ml/min. The left atrial vent is clamped. The head end of the patient is raised a little. Supportive bypass with an empty beating heart is continued for a few minutes to allow the heart to recover its rhythm. When cardiac action appears satisfactory the venous line is partially clamped to fill the heart. Cardiopulmonary bypass is partial at this stage. It is important now to inspect all suture lines carefully to ensure proper haemostasis. Special attention is paid to the posterior aortic anastomosis seen through the transverse sinus and the posterior pulmonary homograft suture line. The left atrial vent may now be removed. When satisfied cardiopulmonary bypass may be discontinued. At this time an infusion of nitroglycerine (0–25 mg/kg.min) is begun and aortic systolic pressure is maintained at 80–90 mm Hg. This is necessary to prevent stretching and tearing of anastomotic lines by high aortic systolic pressure. Again all suture lines are carefully inspected and covered with a small dry sponge placed in the transverse sinus and also anteriorly.

The heart generally takes a few minutes (5–10 min) to regain its normal rhythm and contraction, especially when it is filled. Readjustment of the right coronary artery anastomosis takes places when the aortic pressure is restored. It is best to keep the afterload down (aortic systolic pressure) to let the heart recover fully and to let the anastomotic lines to seal themselves. This may take form 15–20 min after cardiopulmonary bypass is discontinued. When satisfied, heparin is reversed and haemostasis and decannulation are completed. If possible the pleural flap is used to cover the heart anteriorly using interrupted sutures.

Two atrial and two ventricular temporary epicardial pacing wires are placed for rhythm control in the postoperative period. A transesophageal echocardiography is performed to assess autograft and left ventricular function. Inotropic support is rarely required and is best avoided to keep the aortic pressure under control. Systolic hypertension in the postoperative period is avoided (to reduce anastomotic leaks) by an infusion of nitroglycerine.

Results

This is a complex operation. When performed well, it can be done with the same risk as isolated aortic valve replacement, less than 3% operative mortality. The long-term results, however, are far superior to any other procedure for aortic valve replacement. The risk of reoperation at 20 years is less than 5%. The causes may be autograft dilatation, infective endocarditis. Structural valve deterioration is almost absent. Reoperation may also be required for right ventricular outflow tract obstruction. This is more likely in relatively young patients. The use of an appropriate cryopreserved pulmonary homograft can reduce this to less than 10% at 20 years. In the author's experience in 150 patients there has been no reoperation for right ventricular outflow tract at 10 years.

Some caution must be exercised in selection of patients. This operation is contraindicated in young (under 35) rheumatic heart disease patients especially if they have additional mitral valve lesions as well.

It is best avoided in elderly patients (more than 60 years) because of likelihood of atherosclerotic disease of the aorta, coronary and cerebral vessels. In addition, tissue valves provide the best option in this age group.

Suggested Reading

1 Abraham S, Joshi R, Kumar AS. Transaortic double valve replacement with chordal preservation. Texas Heart Inst J 2002 ; 29(2):133-35.

2 Al-Halees Z, Kumar N, Gallo R, Gometza B, Duran CMG. Pulmonary autograft for aortic valve replacement in rheumatic disease: a caveat. Ann. Thorac Surg 1995; 60:S172-6.

3 Barratt-Boyes BG. Aortic allograft valve implantation: freehand or root replacement ? J. Card Surg 1994;9 (Suppl 2):196-7.

4 Barratt-boyes BG. Homograft aortic valve replacement in aortic incompetence and stenosis. Thorax 1964;19: 131-50.

5 Barratt-Boyes BG. Invited commentary on Choudhary et al. J.Cardiac Surg. 1998:13;8.

6 Carmichael MJ, Cooley DA, Favor AS. Aortic and mitral valve replacement through a single transverse aortotomy: a useful approach in difficult mitral valve exposure. Texas Heart Inst J 1983;10:415-9.

7 Chambers JC, Somerville J, Stone S, Ross DN. Pulmonary autograft procedure for aortic valve disease: long–term results of the pioneer series. Circulation 1997;96:2206-14

8 Choudhary SK, Govil A, Kumar AS. Ross Procedure : Aortic Valve Replacement with Pulmonary Autograft. Ind. J. Thorac Cardiovasc Surg 2001:17;243-257.

9 Choudhary SK , Govil A, KumarAS. Ross Procedure : Aortic valve replacement with pulmonary autograft. J. Thorac Cardiovasc Surg 2001;14:243-57.

10 Choudhary SK, Mathur A, Chander H, Saxena A, Dogra TD, Venugopal P, Kumar AS. Aortic valve replacement with Biological Substitute. J.Cardiac Surg. 1998:13, 1-8.

11 Choudhary SK, Mathur A, Sharma R, Saxena A, Chopra P, Roy R, Kumar AS. Pulmonary autograft : should it be used in young patients with Rheumatic Disease? J. Thorac. Cardiovasc. Surg 1999; 118(3):483-90 discussion 490-1.

12 Crawford ES, Coselli JS. Marfan's syndrome: combined composite valve graft replacement of the aortic root and trans aortic mitral valve replacement. Ann. Thorac Surg 1988;45:296-302.

13 Duran C, Kumar N, Gometza B, Halees ZA. Aortic valve reconstruction. Ann. Thorac Surg 1991;52:447-54.

14 Duran CMG. Reconstructive techniques for rheumatic aortic valve disease.J Cardiac Surg 1988;3:23-29.

15 Elkins RC. The Ross operation : a 12-year experience. Ann. Thorac Surg 1999;68(3):S14-8.

16 kouchoukos NT, Masetti P, Nickerson NJ, Castner CF, Shannon WD, Davila-Roman VG. The Ross procedure: long-term clinical and echocardiographic follow-up. Ann. Thorac Surg 2004;78:773-81.

17 Kumar AS, Gundane P. Aortic Valve Repair : Technique and Results. Asian Cardiovascular and Thoracic Annals, 1994;2:75-77.

18 Kumar AS, Rao PN. Restoration of Pliability to Mitral leaflets during reconstruction. J.Heart Valve Dis 1995;4:251-253.

19 Kumar AS, Rao PN, Dharmapuram AK, Chander H, Trehan H. Pulmonary Autograft Aortic Valve Replace-

ment : Early experience with the Ross Procedure. Texas Heart Inst J 1995; 22(2): 177-9.

20 Kumar AS, Rao PN, Trehan H. A technique to prevent bleeding after Ross Procedure. J. Heart Valve Dis 1995; 4(4): 405-6.

21 Kumar AS, Talwar S, Mohapatra R, Saxena A, Singh R. Aortic valve replacement with the pulmonary autograft: Mid-term results. Ann. Thorac Surg 2005; 80(2):488-94.

22 Kumar AS, Talwar S, Saxena A, Singh R. Ross procedure in Rheumatic Aortic Valve Disease. J. Thorac Cardiovasc Surg 2006;29:156-161.

23 Kumar AS. The Ross operation in rheumatic valve disease. Cir Cardiov 2005 ; 12(2) : 121-2.

24 Kumar AS, Saxena A. Intraoperative transoesophageal echocardiography in aortic valve surgery. Indian Heart J 2000;52(1):50-3.

25 Kumar N, Prabhakar G, Gometza B, Al-Halees Z, Duran CM. The Ross procedure in the young rheumatic population:early clinical and echo-cardiographic profile. J. Heart Valve Dis 1993;2:376-9.

26 O'Brien MF, Finney RS, Stafford G, et al. Root replacement for all allograft aortic valves: Preferred technique or too radical? Ann. Thorac Surg 1995;60: S87-S91

27 O'Brien MF, Harrocks S, Stafford EG, et al. The homograft aortic valve : a 29-year, 99.3% follow up of 1,022 valve replacement. J Heart Valve Dis 2001;10: 334-44.

28 O'Brien MF, McGiffin DC, Stafford EG, et al. Allograft aortic valve replacement : Long-term comparative clinical analysis of the viable cryopreserved and antibiotic 4-degreees C stored valves. J Card Surg 1991;61(Suppl): 534-543.

29 O'Brien MF, Stafford EG, Gardner MAH, et al. Allograft aortic valve replacement: Long term follow up. Ann. Thorac Surg 1995;60:S65-S70.

30 Oury JH, Angell WW, Eddy AC, Cleveland JC. Pulmonary autograft-past, present, and future. J. Heart Valve Dis. 1993;2:365-75.

31 Rao PN, Kumar AS. Aortic Valve Replacement through Right Thoracotomy. Texas Heart Inst J 1993; 20(4): 307-8.

32 Ross D, Jackson M, Davies J. The pulmonary autograft—a permanent aortic valve. Eur J Cardiothorac Surg 1992;6:113-6.

33 Ross D. Technique of aortic valve replacement with a homograft: orthotopic replacement. Ann. Thorac Surg 1991;52:154-6.

34 Ross DN. Homograft replacement of the aortic valve. Lancet 1962;2:487-93.

35 Ross DN. Replacement of aortic and mitral valves with a pulmonary autograft. Lancet 1967;2:956-8.

36 Spencer FC, Doyle EF, Danilowicz DA, Bahnson HT, Weldon CS. Long-term evaluation of aortic valvuloplasty for aortic insufficiency and ventricular septal defect. J. Thorac Cardiovasc Surg. 1973 Jan;65(1):15-31.

37 Talwar S, Mohapatra R, Saxena A, Singh R, Kumar AS. Aortic homograft : A suitable substitute for aortic valve replacement. Ann. Thorac Surg 2005;80(3):832-8.

38 Talwar S, Pradeep KK, Gulati GS, Kumar AS. Right coronary ostial transection during aortic valve replacement: Technique of reconstruction. Ind J.of Thorac and Cardiovasc Surg 2005;21:00-01.

39 Talwar S, Saikrishna C, Saxena A, Kumar AS. Aortic valve repair for rheumatic aortic valve disease. Ann. Thorac Surg 2005;79(6):1921-5.

40 Trusler GA, Moes CAF, Kidd BSL. Repair of ventricular septal defect with aortic insufficiency. J Thorac Cardiovasc Surg 1973;66:394-403.

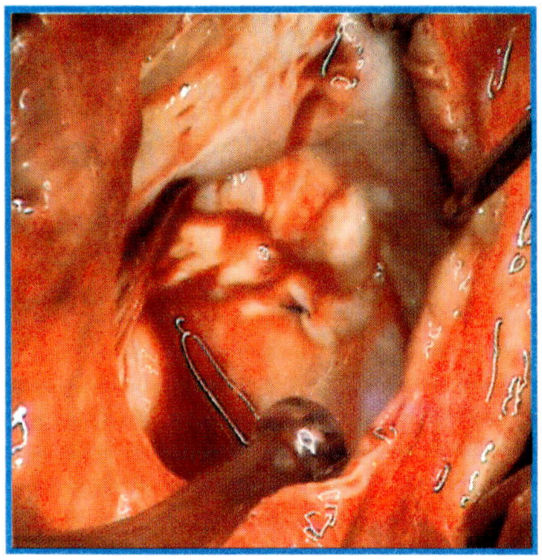

3

The Tricuspid Valve

Anatomy

The tricuspid valve has unique anatomical relations. Located anteriorly in the cardiac fibrous skeleton, it has three well recognised cusps. As seen at surgery it is related to the aortic valve between 7 to 9 O'clock positions. On the septal side it forms one side of the triangle of Koch between the 4 O'clock to 7 O'clock positions, the apex of which is at the 7 O'clock position where the penetrating bundle (bundle of His) enters the septum. The base of the triangle is formed by the opening of the coronary sinus. The 9 O'clock to 4 O'clock anterior D-shaped annulus can be perilously close to the right coronary artery. For the surgeon it is best to keep away from the septal tricuspid annulus and any sutures placed in this area are best placed through the base of the septal cusp.

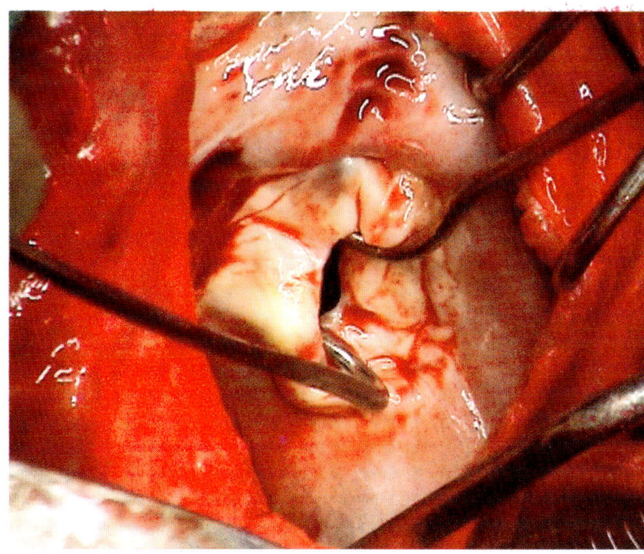

Fig. 3.1: Severe tricuspid stenosis.

Physiology

The tricuspid valve opens and closes earlier than the mitral valve. The annulus is more dynamic than the mitral annulus and collapses more than 30% of its diameter in systolic. Severe tricuspid regurgitation can, therefore, result from high pressure in the right ventricle, as in pulmonary hypertension (functional tricuspid regurgitation). Acquired tricuspid stenosis is almost always due to rheumatic heart disease.

Pathology

Tricuspid stenosis occurs in rheumatic heart disease and can reduce the tricuspid orifice to less than 1 cm^2 (Fig. 3.1). However, gradients of 2–3 mmHg denote significant stenosis of the valve. Fusion usually manifests at the commissures of the septal cusp with the anterior and posterior cusps. There is usually thickening of the cusps as well. Tricuspid regurgitation in such patients can be severe and is termed organic tricuspid regurgitation in contrast to functional tricuspid regurgitation seen in pulmonary arterial hypertension. The tricuspid valve is also the seat of vegetation and fungal endocarditis in intravenous drug abusers. Tricuspid valve disease (except endocarditis) is almost never seen in isolation and is always accompanied by mitral and /or aortic valve disease.

Tricuspid Valvotomy

Tricuspid valvotomy is indicated in patients with severe tricuspid stenosis. The approach in such patients is through the right atrium even for the mitral lesion.

A midsternotomy or right anterior thoracotomy may be used. Cardiopulmonary bypass is established with bicaval and aortic cannulation. The superior vena cava and inferior vena cava are taped. Aorta is cross clamped and cardioplegia is infused into the aortic root. It is important to vent the left atrium if there is mitral regurgitation and to pass an instrument such as a ligature carrier into the mitral valve if there is mitral stenosis in order to avoid distension of the left ventricle. When cardioplegia has been delivered, the caval tapes are snugged. The right atrium is opened from the right atrial appendage towards the inferior vena cava with an incision parallel to the atrioventricular groove. Stay sutures are placed on the right atrial wall for retraction. The fossa ovalis is identified and an incision is made. The left atrium is emptied of all blood. This septal incision is extended towards the inferior vena cava. The medical flap is retracted by two small Mayo retractors bringing into view the mitral valve. The mitral procedure is then completed (Fig. 3.2).

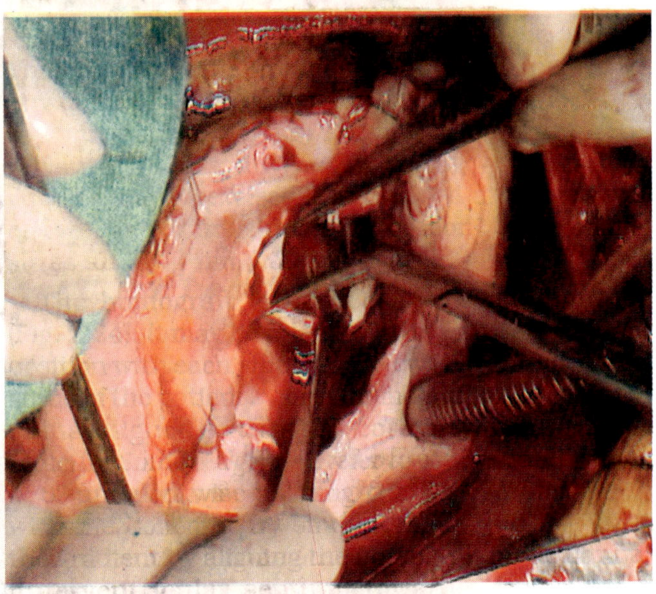

Fig. 3.2: Tricuspid valvotomy. The commissure between the anterior and the septal cusps in being incised.

The anterior wall is gently retracted with a Cooley tricuspid retractor, bringing the tricuspid valve into view. The cusps and commissures are identified. Two curved hooks are placed under the anterior and septal cusps for gentle traction. This will highlight the fused commissure which is now incised with a no. 11 blade from the orifice towards the annulus. A similar incision is made in the fused commissure between the septal and posterior cusps. This will in effect provide a bicuspid valve with one anterior (and posterior) and one septal cusp. The third commissure need not be incised as it rarely interferes with function even when fused. The valve is now tested for competence by injecting saline into the right ventricle. Generally there is important tricuspid regurgitation which requires correction.

Tricuspid Valve Repair

Tricuspid regurgitation is most often caused by pulmonary arterial hypertension in mitral valve disease (functional tricuspid regurgitation) or due to rheumatic involvement of the tricuspid valve itself. It may also be due to infective endocarditis.

A repair procedure is preferred because a suitable substitute for the bicuspid valve is not yet available. A De Vega type of repair is the most effective and popular technique. The Carpentier technique involves implantation of an annuloplasty ring (Fig. 3.3).

De Vega Tricuspid Repair

The tricuspid valve is exposed as described earlier. A 3-0 polypropylene pledgeted double arm suture is used. The first needle passes 2–3 mm away from the tricuspid annulus beginning at the 4 O'clock position upwards gathering the right atrial wall in a purse-string fashion. This is continued anticlockwise and ends at the 7 O'clock position on the left of the tricuspid valve. The second needle also begins at the 4 O'clock position gathering the right atrial wall parallel to the first suture and about 1–2 mm away from it and ends at the 7 O'clock position. Both needles are now passed through a Teflon pledget. The suture is now tightened until about 25–30% of the tricuspid annulus circumference is reduced. In order to avoid tricuspid stenosis two fingers of the surgeon may be kept in the tricuspid orifice during this annuloplasty. The handle of the Cooley mitral valve retractor is a good substitute and can be held in the tricuspid orifice while tightening and tying the suture. The suture is now tied. The competence is checked by injecting saline into the right ventricle. If satisfactory the Teflon pledget is fixed with a 5-0 polypropylene suture at this point.

Carpentier Annuloplasty

The tricuspid valve is sized using the special annuloplasty sizers. An appropriate sized ring is chosen. It is sutured to the tricuspid annulus using 3-0 or 4-0 braided sutures using a horizontal mattress technique. Roughly 12–15 such sutures may be required. The sutures on the septal side are taken from the right ventricular side out into the right atrial side through the base of the septal cusp. The tricuspid annuloplasty ring is also incomplete

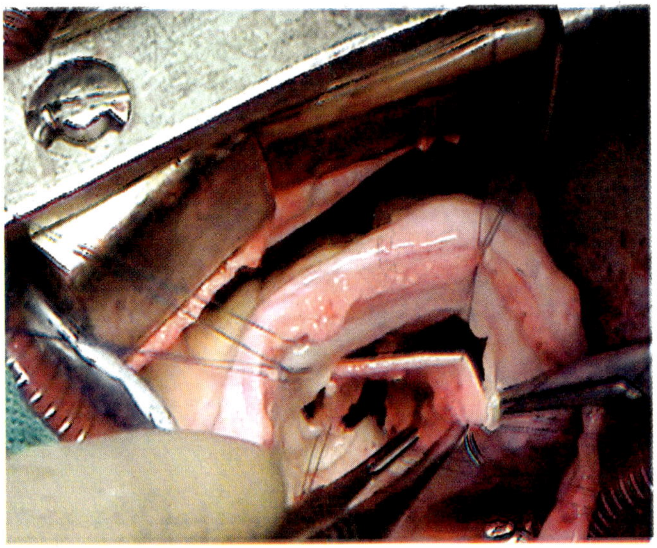

Fig. 3.3: Reconstruction of the tricuspid valve with autologous pericardium.

in the region of the bundle of His where no sutures are placed. All these double-armed needles are passed through the annuloplasty ring. The ring is lowered and all sutures are pulled taut. The valve is tested for competence. If satisfactory, the sutures are tied.

A flexible ring may also be used (Duran, Cosgrove) and deformed to fit the shape and size of the tricuspid valve. Also a Pugh Masanna ring which can reduce the annulus after fixation may also be used. The ultimate aim is to abolish the tricuspid regurgitation without producing stenosis.

Tricuspid Valve Replacement

Tricuspid valve replacement should be considered a last (desperate) option when repair is impossible. This is because the mortality is very high (nearly 25–30%) and a suitable substitute is not currently available. Mechanical valves fail uniformly because of the low pressure system. Bioprosthetic valves have better survival and function but tend to degenerate sooner than in the mitral position. Some recent interest in mitral homografts as a substitute appears feasible.

An appropriate stented bioprosthesis (porcine/ pericardial) is chosen. The valve orientation should ensure that one stent is at 9 O'clock position . The prosthesis is anchored with 2-0 braided sutures placed in horizontal mattress fashion. The sutures must avoid the bundle of His. The tricuspid leaflets are not excised but are retained to buttress the suture line especially on the septal aspect. Following replacement the right atrium is closed and care is taken during deairing not to distort the bio-prosthesis struts or to injure the right ventricular wall.

Results

The immediate haemodynamic results of tricuspid valvotomy and tricuspid valve repair are excellent. Mortality is dependent on the primary mitral/aortic lesion, left ventricular function and presence of hepatic/renal dysfunction. Mortality is usually in 8–10% range and most patients have a difficult or stormy postoperative course. They require inotropic and respiratory support. Hepatic and renal failure are higher in this group of patients. Tricuspid valve replacement has a high early mortality of 25–30% and poor long-term results due to structural valve degeneration.

Suggested Reading

1 Carpentier A, Deloche A, Hanania G, Forman J, Sellier P, Piwnica A, Dubost C, McGoon DC. Surgical management of acquired tricuspid valve disease. J. Thorac Cardiovasc Surg. 1974 Jan;67(1):53-65.

2 Grondin P, Meere C, Limet R, Lopez-Bescos L, Delcan JL, Rivera R. Carpentier's annulus and De Vegas annuloplasty. The end of the tricuspid challenge. J. Thorac Cardiovasc Surg. 1975 Nov;70(5):852-61.

3 Kulshrestha P, Das B, Iyer KS, Kumar AS, Sharma ML,Rao IM, Kaul U, Srivastava S, Venugopal P. Surgical experience with disease of the tricuspid valve : Cross sectional and Doppler Echocardiographic evaluation following DeVega repair. Int.J.Cardiol. 23 : 19-26, 1989.

4 Kumar AS, Iyer KS, Chopra P. Quadrivalvular heart disease. Int. J. Cardiol.1985;7(1):66-69.

5 Talwar S, Jayanthkumar HV, Sharma G, Kumar AS. Quadrivalvular rheumatic heart disease. Int. J. Cardiol. 2006 Jan 4;106(1):117-8.

6 Victor S, Nayak VM. Tricuspid valve is bicuspid. Ann. Thrac. Surg. 2006;69:1989-90.

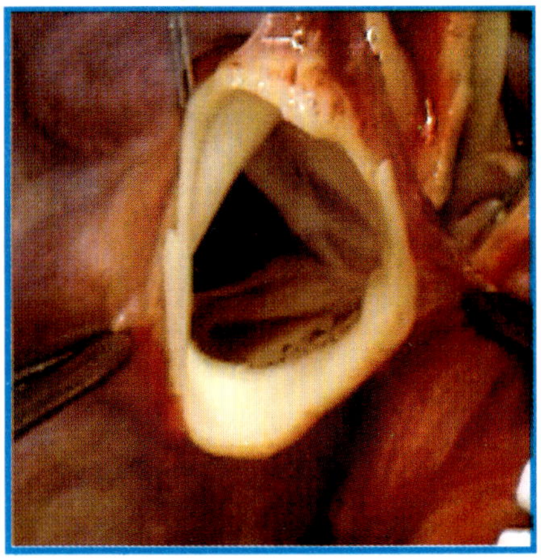

4 The Pulmonary Valve

Anatomy

This is an identical twin of the semilunar aortic valve. It is usually located 5–10 mm distal form the plane of the aortic valve and has one anterior and two posterior sinuses. The pulmonary valve is capable of withstanding systemic pressure loading (as in severe pulmonary arterial hypertension) without loss of function.

Physiology

The pulmonary valve normally closes after the aortic valve. It is quite adaptive and can accommodate both higher pressure and flows. Mild to moderate regurgitation does not produce significant symptoms in isolation. However, long standing pulmonary regurgitation can and does result in right ventricular dysfunction.

Pathology

Pulmonary valve stenosis is almost always congenital. It is no longer a surgical problem since balloon dilatation is extremely successful, cost effective and avoids major surgery.

Chronic rheumatic valvulitis of the pulmonary valve is rare and is usually associated with stenotic lesion of the mitral, aortic and tricuspid valves. It should be suspected and looked for if the other three valves are stenotic.

Pulmonary Valvotomy

Pulmonary valvotomy is indicated (currently) only with associated other congenital defects such as atrial septal defect, ventricular septal defect and tetrology of Fallot. It is also indicated in quadrivalvular rheumatic heart disease. The technique involves opening the pulmonary artery by a transverse incision under cardiopulmonary bypass and incising the commissures under direct vision. The orifice is now dilated by passing a Hegar dilator into the right ventricle through the pulmonary valve orifice. One must look for and divide any obstructing muscle bands in the right ventricular outflow tract to avoid a residual gradient. Mild to moderate degrees of pulmonary regurgitation are usually well tolerated and does not require replacement.

Pulmonary Valve Replacement

This is indicated in patients undergoing Ross procedures (I and II) and in patients who have severe pulmonary regurgitation following corrective surgery for tetrology of Fallot, or for absent pulmonary valve syndrome. The pulmonary (or aortic) homograft is the best substitute. One may use a more easily available pulmonary xenograft valve (porcine). The technique has been described earlier with the Ross procedure.

Results

Pulmonary valvotomy does not add to the mortality in patients with quadrivalvar rheumatic heart disease. In congenital pulmonary stenosis surgery can be accomplished (if necessary) without mortality and with excellent long-term results.

Pulmonary valve replacement in infants children and adolescents (with a homograft) generally requires a reoperation within 5–10 years. In older patients a 10% reoperation rate for right ventricular outflow tract obstruction may be required at 20 years following a Ross procedure.

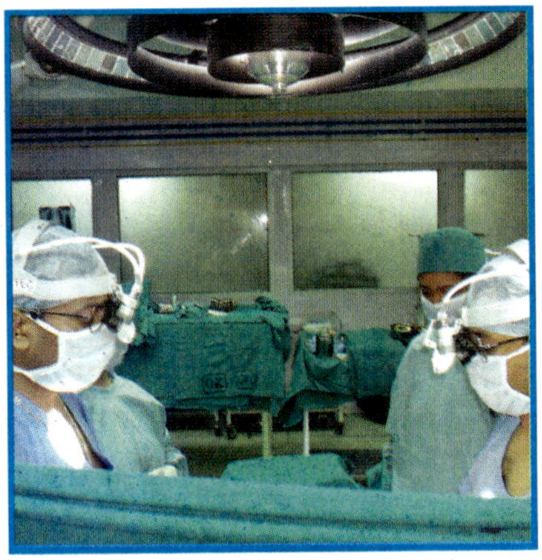

5 Good Surgical Etiquette

Nature thrives on imperfection. No human is perfect as everyone is born with a flaw, an imperfection with which a full and productive life is possible. Therefore when performing surgery try not to achieve a perfect result. It usually results in the most bizarre and unusual complication.

In surgery you must assist nature. Do not try to do better than nature. Nature is resilient and forgiving. It will adjust to minor imperfections.

It is no longer fashionable to be the fastest surgeon. Experienced surgeons perform the same operation efficiently and effortlessly perhaps faster than the fastest surgeon. Their movements are orchestrated perfectly. They do not waste movements or waste their energy on the inconsequential steps.

Cardiac surgery is the best example of team effort. To give the patient the best you must solicit and bring out the best in others. Be generous with your compliments, appreciate a new and good idea from others, and thank all when your surgery is done. You are nothing if your anaesthetist, assistant, nurse or perfusionist are not in tune with you. A simple operation can easily become a disaster.

Be calm and patient, you can neither give nor takeaway life. It is for you to perform a good operation. The result will take care of itself.

Your patient is your best advertisement. Smile and exchange pleasantries. Communication at the soul level cures half the problem. Take a positive attitude in everything. Do not fret and frown when things are not going your way, take a break, divert your attention from the immediate problem, the solution will pop up almost like magic. Focus on the solution and not on the problem.

What you have learned is useless, unless you can give it to others. Teach; those who learn from you will cherish the knowledge. What you leave behind when you go must be for forever, because you are temporary. What you teach will benefit the patient, who comes to you trustingly.

Earn respect. It is the only commodity worth earning. Everything else is available for a price.

Never refuse to help a colleague, junior or assistant who is in trouble. Your help can save an innocent victim. Bury your ego or bury your patient. All others will survive and thrive.

During surgery the greatest calamity also has a solution, you have a very short time to find it. Do not spend your time or energy and lose sight of the obvious.

Be receptive to new ideas and change. Adapt them to your local conditions. Technology transfer must be tempered with an understanding of local conditions. Everything they do is not the best for you.

In the operation theatre everyone looks up to the surgeon. Wear your best attitude and you will get the best from others as well.

Do not curb creativity, encourage it: It is the essence of life, without creativity we will all be in an asylum.

When you watch a surgeon performing with ease, be sure that it has taken him hard work for years to reach there. You cannot acquire it simply by watching him.

Cardiac surgery requires craftsmanship. Everyone can make a chair, only a skilled craftsman makes it comfortable and long-lasting.

Darkness of the mind and illumination of the patient cannot achieve good results. The most powerful light or lens cannot show you the defect if you do not know where to look for it.

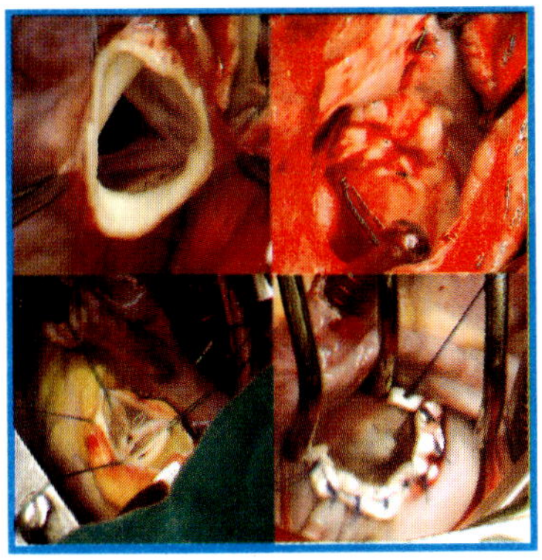

Appendices

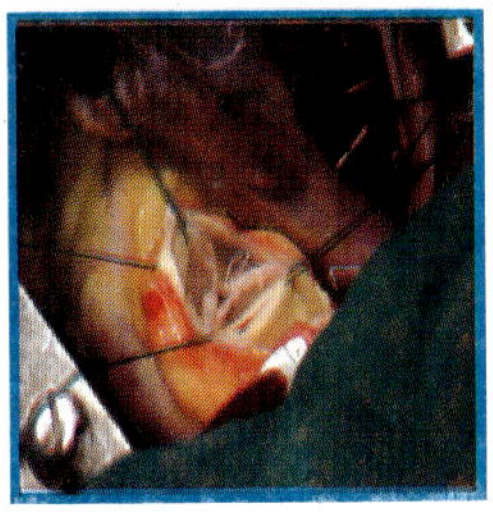

Appendix I

Aortic Valve Replacement

Choice of Aortic Valve Substitute Based on Aortic annulus diameter, Age and Etiology

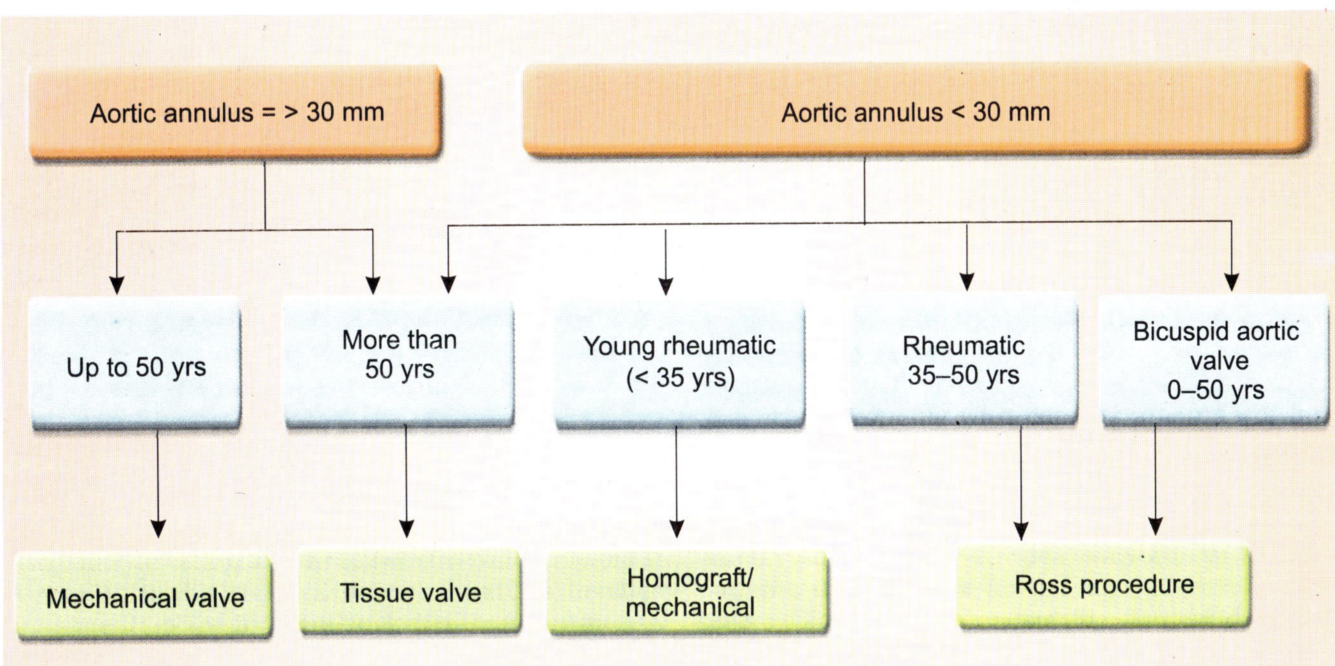

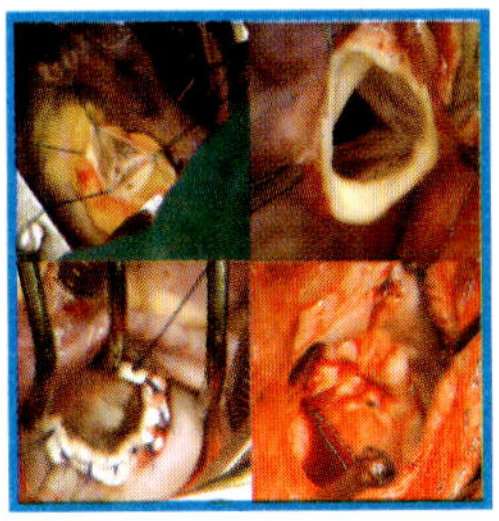

Appendix II

Valve Bank

Donor Selection

No sepsis, infections, or communicable disease; no neoplasm other than carcinoma of skin, in-situ carcinoma of the uterus, or an intracranial neoplasm; no evidence of serious illness of unknown etiology; no drug abuse, poisoning, prolonged steroid treatment, systemic viremia, or fungemia. No history of previous cardiac surgery, hypertension, valvular disease, bacterial endocarditis, rheumatic fever, or untreated active pulmonary disease; no cardiac or chest wall trauma with prolonged closed chest resuscitation. Age range from newborn to 50 years. Time limit for procuring the heart; within 24 hours of death.

Procurement

The pericardium is opened in the midline. The ascending aorta, aortic arch, and the proximal 2 to 3 cm of the arch vessels are dissected free. The superior vena cava and inferior vena cava are dissected and transected. The heart is everted and the pulmonary veins are divided taking care not to open the pericardium posteriorly. The right and left pulmonary arteries are dissected as far as possible and transected. Finally, the aorta is transected distally as far as possible. The heart is removed and rinsed in cold saline to remove blood. It is then packaged in 500 mL of cold saline at 4° C in a sterile double bag and transported to the storage area adjacent to the operating theaters. The donors' blood samples obtained at autopsy are tested for blood group (ABO and Rh), human immunodeficiency virus, hepatitis, and venereal disease.

Dissection

Dissection is carried out in a sterile area using an aseptic technique within the confines of a laminar flow hood. The heart is removed from the transport solution and placed in a sterile basin containing 1.5 L saline solution at 4° C. The pulmonary artery is separated from the aorta. Then the right ventricular cavity is entered anteriorly and by circumferential dissection the pulmonary valve and pulmonary artery are separated from the right ventricle. The roof of the left atrium is incised to expose the mitral valve. The dissection is carried down along the aorto-mitral curtain between the left atrium and the posterior wall of the aorta with a pair of scissors. On reaching a level about 3 mm above the mitral annulus, the aorto-mitral curtain is stabbed with a No. 15 blade. After inspecting the aortic valve, the incision is extended laterally and anteriorly on both sides and the aortic valve conduit is obtained. Thereafter, the free wall of the right ventricle is incised, the interventricular septum is incised vertically through the right ventricular cavity, and the left ventricular cavity is entered. Finally, the papillary muscles are divided near their bases and the mitral valve is dissected free from the atrial wall. The aortic and pulmonary homografts are sized with a conical sizer and labeled.

The anterior mitral leaflet may be retained with the aortic homograft, the incision in this situation divides the chordae to the anterior mitral leaflet and then proceeds circumferentially.

Sterilization

The following antibiotics are added to 1 L of sterile filtered nutrient tissue culture medium (Hanks' balanced salt solution):

cefoxitin 250 mg
lincomycin 120 mg
polymyxin B 100 mg
vancomycin 50 mg
nystatin one million units

HEPES buffer is added to maintain the pH between 6.6 and 7.0. Approximately 100 ml of sterile solution is added to each homograft for storage at 4° C. Antibiotic preserved homografts are best used within 40 days.

Microbiological Procedures

A sample for culture is taken from the cold saline used to transport the heart. Tricuspid valve tissue is sent for fungal and bacterial cultures. The antibiotic solution used to preserve the homograft is filtered through a 0.45 μm filter using an aseptic technique. The filter paper is incubated in thioglycolate broth at 7° C for 7 days and then plated aerobically onto trypticase soya agar. The growth plates are read after two days of incubation at 37° C. Fungal cultures are evaluated after intervalvs of one week and three weeks. The eventual use of the homograft is based on confirmation of tissue sterility.

Cryopreservation

Cryopreservation is begun immediately following the antibiotic incubation period of 48 hours. However, homografts obtained from transplant recipients are not treated with antibiotics and are used or cryopreserved directly. The homograft is removed from the antibiotic container in a sterile manner, rinsed in fresh medium, and packaged with enough freezing solution to produce a total volume of 100 ml. At the time of packaging, cultures are obtained of all the solutions. The valves and the freezing solution are packed in sterile plastic bags, the air is evacuated, and the bags are heat sealed in an aluminium container. The freezing medium used consisted of RPMI 1640 tissue culture medium. (Rose Park Memorial Institute tissue culture medium no. 1640) with 10% fetal calf serum amended with dimethyl sulfoxide to a 10% concentration. The tissue is frozen at a rate of 1° C per minute in a Kryo 10 controlled rate freezer (Planer Products Ltd, Sunbury-on-Thames, Middlesex, UK) to a temperature of – 40° C, then rapidly cooled to – 150° C. The homograft is then transferred for permanent storage in vapor phase liquid nitrogen between– 150° C and – 190° C in a XLC 500 vacuum insulated Dewar flask (Minnesota Valley Engineering Inc., Bloomington, MN, USA).

Thawing

Before implantation, the cryopreserved homograft needs to be thawed for approximately 20 minutes in a water bath at a temperature of 37° C to 42° C within the plastic bag. The homograft is than agitated twice for 3 minutes in a solution of RPMI tissue culture medium and 10% fetal calf serum to remove the cryopreservative. Subsequently, the homograft is transferred to 50 ml of the recipient's heparinized blood before implantation.

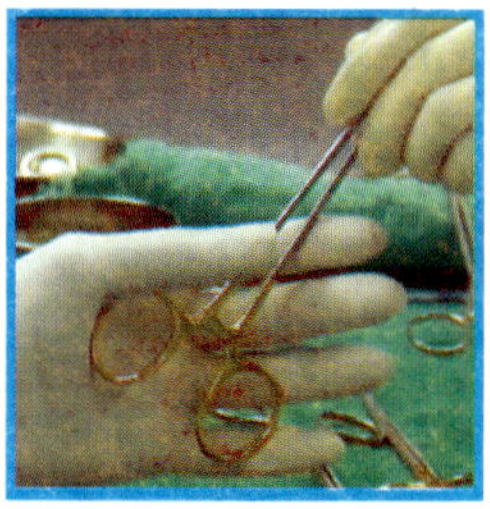

Appendix III

A Note on Handling Surgical Instruments

In cardiovascular surgery the surgeon needs to master the use of two very essential and important instruments. These are a pair of vascular (autraumatic) forceps in the left hand and a needle holder in the right hand (Figs A1, A2, A3).

Without changing the grip on the needle holder the surgeon can rotate the needle on its axis for either forehand or backhand suture passage.

The author believes that mastering these two instruments helps in ease of suturing, with increased speed and elegance. For the observer these movements appear simple but need mastering by practice.

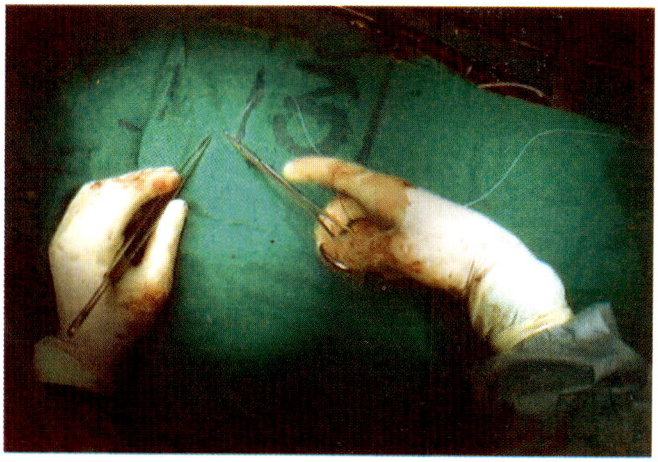

Fig. A2: The relative positions of the hands with the vascular forceps. The right hand position is for a forehand pass of the needle.

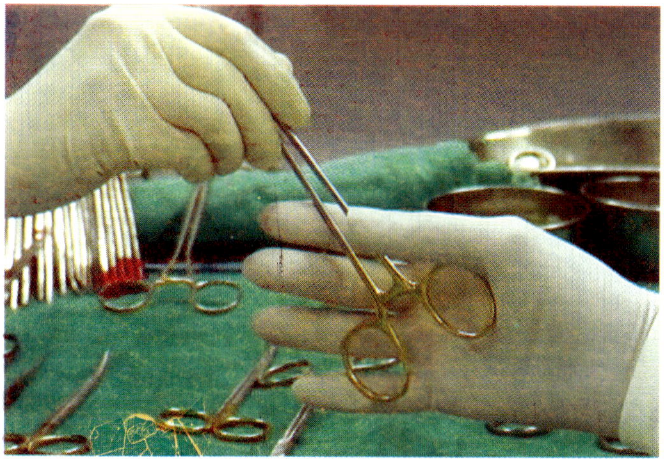

Fig. A1: The scrub nurse hands the needle holder to the surgeon.

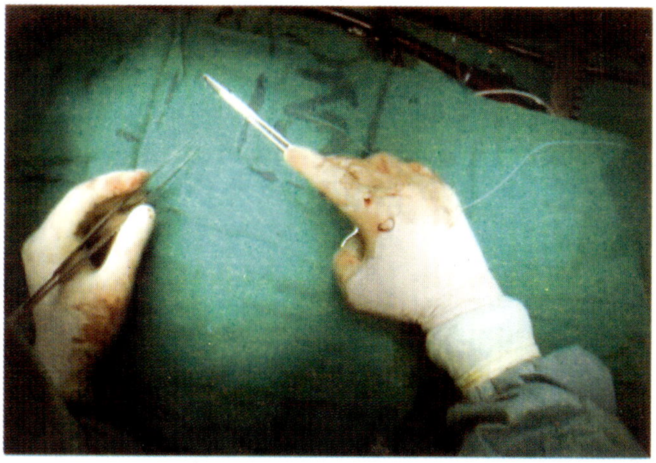

Fig. A3: The same grip of the needle holder but different position of the hand for a backhand pass of the suture. In both the figures note the position of the thumb.

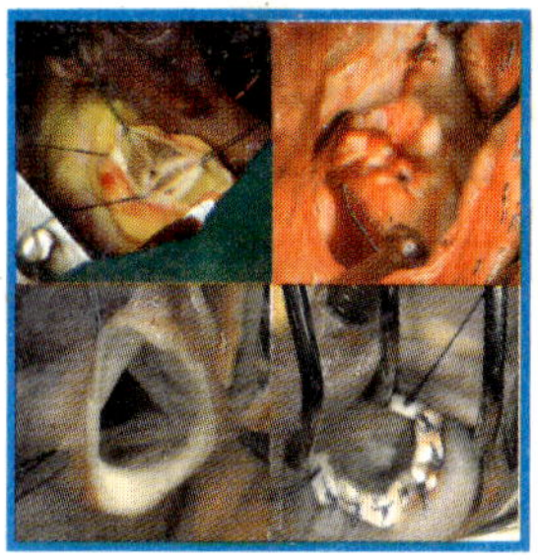

Index